AF239665

Breaking new ground in diagnosis and therapy in veterinary medicine

Bioresonance therapy: so simple – so ingenious

Dr. med. vet. Jochen Becker

Breaking new ground in diagnosis and therapy in veterinary medicine

Bioresonance therapy:
so simple – so ingenious

Dr. med. vet. Jochen Becker

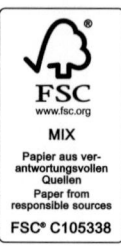

© 2013 Jochen Becker
Cover, production and publishing: Books on Demand GmbH, Norderstedt
ISBN 978-3-8482-3231-4

Bibliographic information of the German National Library
The German National Library lists this publication in the German National Biblio-
graphy; detailed bibliographic data are available on the internet at http://dnb.d-nb.de

Table of contents

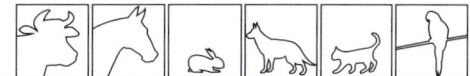

How I got involved in bioresonance therapy

When I completed my veterinary medicine studies at Hanover University of Veterinary Medicine and received my veterinary degree, I was absolutely convinced that I was able to treat and cure animals professionally with the help of rapidly developing medical science. Everything was so plain and coherent: there was a biochemical explanation for every disease and for what was happening when and where in the organism, and what was causing the particular symptom. We obviously simply needed the right antidote and the animal would be well again. However, I found that in many cases I did not achieve the result I had hoped for.

I had also experienced the same in my own medical history. At the age of 5 I was most probably one of the first patients to be examined for various allergens in a university hospital in North Rhine Westphalia with an extensive allergy diagnosis obtained with the help of a prick test on my back.

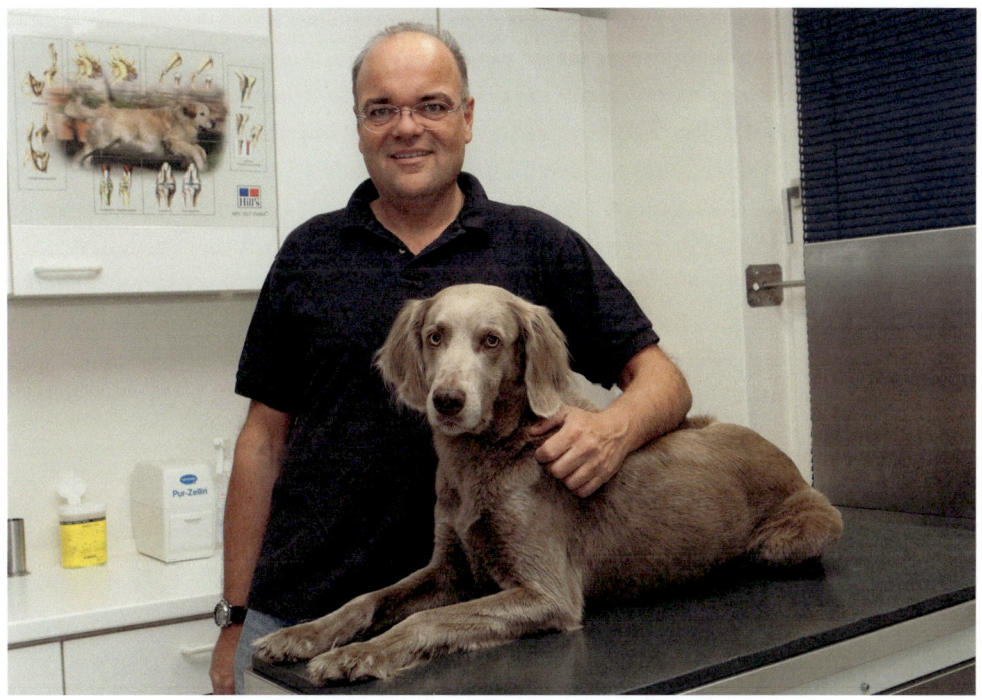

The author Dr. Jochen Becker with his Weimaraner bitch Camill von Stemmer.

This was followed by annual allergen-desensitizing procedures – a total of 13. Although the doctors hoped to be able to treat my seasonal allergies, instead they constantly got worse. Despite this treatment, no relief was possible without additional cortisone compounds which I had to take from the age of 5. But since I was a conventional medical practitioner, this was all comprehensible to me. And so was the allergic asthma that appeared when I was 24.

Further health problems occurred: back pain due to a stenosis of the spinal cord over 4 lumbar vertebrae, which nobody was able to get a grip on with any kind of conventional treatment. But I always tried to remain calm, telling myself that there was simply no medication on the market yet and that I just had to hold out long enough until science was able to offer a cure with an "anti-symptom compound". And until then I had "my cortisone" and "my asthma spray" to get along.

When I finished my veterinary studies I was so convinced of what I was doing that each client who entered my practice and told me about naturopathic treatment methods was quickly silenced, if not shown the door. However, this changed completely, if quite by accident. My son who was 7 at the time asked me to go cycling with him regularly. However, this was rather difficult for me due to my considerable "spare tyre". I tried to secretly get back in shape and to lose weight. However this was very frustrating as I was not able to cycle more than 10 km a day – any further was simply impossible. So I went in good faith to my family practitioner and asked him what I could to do build up stamina. He did a long-term ECG, a stress ECG and checked my blood. Fortunately all the results were normal so that the doctor was convinced that, due to my 40 year medical history with cortisone, hypertension, lipometabolism problems and my back problems, I simply had to live with the fact that I was getting old. I was 44 at the time! However, this kept bothering me so that I started searching the internet for a practitioner who might give me a different opinion. I quickly found a sports physician who was also an anaesthetist.

At my first appointment he asked me what my problem was. I told me my story and he asked me something I had never expected: "Why?" I responded "What do you mean – why"?" He simply said: "All you have told me so far are just symptoms but why do you have all this?" I replied "Well, my father and my mother…." - "No, no", he said, "I want to know why you manifest all these indications. There must be a reason for these symptoms." At the time I still questioned his opinion but, while I was there, I agreed to be examined with a bioresonance device. He found all sorts of stresses: intolerances, interference caused by scars, Candida etc. and started to treat me.

I went home rather disbelieving and waited one day. The day after the therapy I climbed on my bike and, believe it or not, I rode 65 km and would have gone even further if I had not become scared of my own body – and if not for an ice cream parlour. Of course I was not cured after one treatment – it took a number of further treatments to finally be symptom-free. But this first treatment made me realize it was worth giving all that I had experienced a second thought and I decided to find out more about bioresonance, which until then I had discounted as complete nonsense with my blinkered conventional medical view.

There were so many patients in my practice with food allergies, recurring lameness, so many with chronic pulmonary diseases or chronic diarrhoea – was there possibly a way to cure them?

So far, I have carried out about 1,100 bioresonance treatments on my patients within 4 years. My practice has changed from a conventional medical practice to a holistic practice and I am no longer prescribing my patients long-term therapy with "anti-symptom treatment" but am finally able to cure them. Don't we, as animal therapists, all have the aim of being able to help and cure? My aim in the practice today is to find the cause of a disease and to cure it and I am happy that my own long and unnecessary medical history has finally put me on track. I hope this book will convince you, too – don't let anything stand in your way as it did me for so many years.

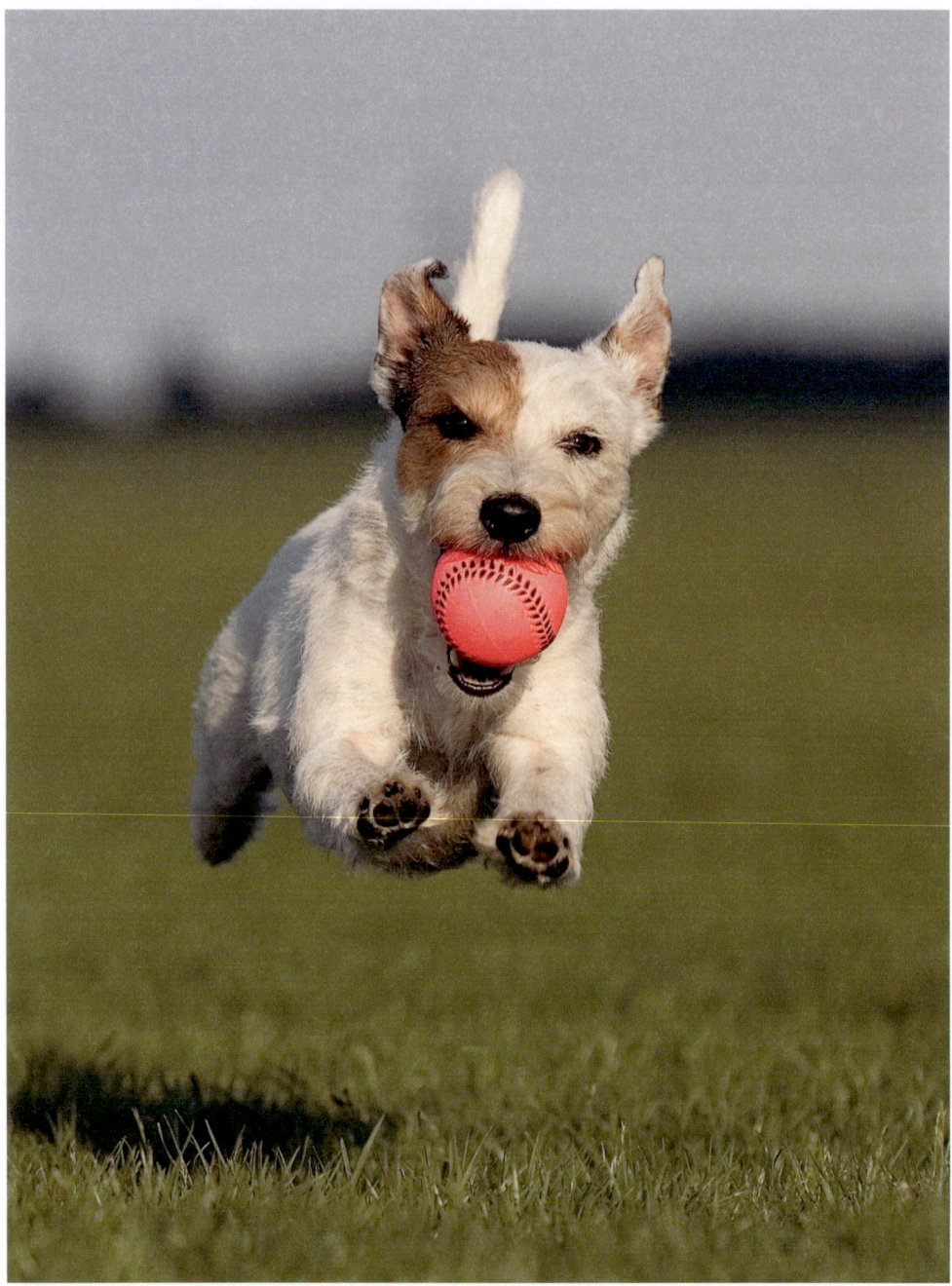

A healthy animal is the aim of successful therapy.

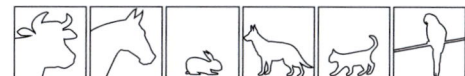

What is bioresonance?

Just like acupuncture, homeopathy and the various energetic cures, bioresonance is a form of regulative or complementary medicine.

Bioresonance exploits the fact that all matter consists of condensed energy and that all matter reflects a frequency pattern. These findings are based on Einstein's general and special theories of relativity which proved, in quantum physics, that each elementary particle can be described as a material particle and as a wave.

A lot of research has been carried out trying to refute or confirm these theories. However our knowledge in this area is not yet complete so that there still exists considerable need for further research.

Conclusive physical evidence about the matter-oscillation issue has not been provided as yet, but it is beyond dispute that there are numerous studies describing the significance of oscillation for an elementary particle and hence, in its entirety, also for the organism. The fact that bioresonance is not yet taught at the various medical universities is mainly because its importance for the specialist field of medicine has not been recognized as yet. And before trying a new but effective method, people prefer to stick to their "defensive stance" according to the principle that "what cannot be must not be".

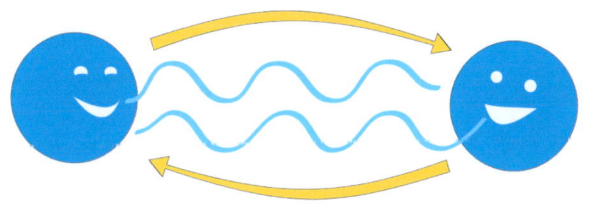

A healthy organism needs working communication between cells.

Eventually each new result in research just adds a further piece to the puzzle so that the next few years will certainly mark a change at the universities too. For instance I am very happy about University Hospital Hamburg Eppendorf opening the "HanseMerkur Centre for Traditional Chinese Medicine" – the first institute for regulatory medicine. And in 2012 the University of Hanover followed with the Medical School running an institute for natural medicine.

After all, this opening of universities is just a logical step in view of the increasing number of chronic diseases that have appeared in the course of recent years where conventional medicine only produces frustrating results. The application of homeopathy at university and clinical facilities was a first step towards complementary medicine and natural medicine. And the knowledge that, in a D potency or higher, a remedy does not contain a single material particle but still causes a reaction, is a clear indication of the efficiency of the oscillation of the original particle in solution.

The Japanese scientist Masura Emoto has marked a milestone in our understanding of this fact by investigating water in different crystalline structures under the electron microscope. Emoto was able to prove that a material that is dissolved in water will always give the water its specific crystalline structure – regardless of the potency. You will, without a doubt, want to know the reason for this fact. It is caused by the so-called cluster structure of water. Due to its chemical structure H_2O, water is weakly positive on 2 poles and weakly negative at the oxygen pole. Therefore it is able to enter a hydrogen bridge relationship with the adjacent water molecule by connecting to the opposed pole and will hence build a cluster structure. When new material is added to this structure, i.e. the water, the existing clusters will locate around this material and will hence create new clusters. These new clusters will still remain even if the original material has been dissolved from the liquid. Each cluster corresponds to a reproducible electromagnetic oscillation which also remains even after the material has been dissolved with the cluster still remaining.

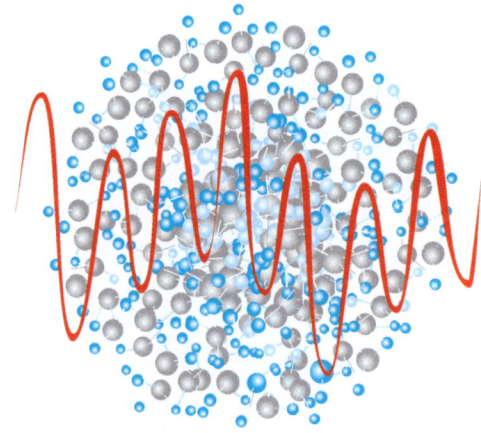

Electromagnetic oscillation made visible.

The electromagnetic oscillation hence remains as the source of information and allows a conclusion to be drawn as regarding the water's memory function.

If we now visualize this idea of the cluster structure as the source of water's memory and information, the step to understanding bioresonance therapy is very small. The body is made up of more than 50% water and all the body's cells are immersed in inter-cellular water. This water absorbs and stores various items of information from metabolic processes, toxins and other agents. The body's self-healing processes are able to eliminate this information to a certain extent and thus avoid possible negative effects. However, a functioning organism requires functioning communication between the cells. The water clusters existing in the body are integrated in this cell communication. If we are able to use bioresonance therapy to rid the water clusters of pathogenic factors with the help of oscillations in the same frequency, we enable the body to let the cells communicate as desired. The body's self-healing processes can be set in motion again.

The bioresonance device

In simple terms the bioresonance device serves to absorb the electromagnetic oscillation patterns from the body of the patient with the help of electrodes and to give them back in modulated form, hence creating healthy oscillation in the body.

These oscillation patterns cannot be captured with simple measurement methods as their field intensity is way below electric background noise. Accordingly measurements can only be carried out in well-equipped laboratories with great effort. However, the body is able to respond to these patterns as they are reflections of its own oscillation pattern in modulated form and as the cells also communicate among each other on this level. This has been proved conclusively by a number of scientific studies.

In contrast to other techniques, Bicom bioresonance therapy hence does not use technically created frequencies but the body's own frequency patterns at the ultrafine energy level. So called entry or input electrodes that are applied to interference fields, pathogenic areas, reflexes or painful zones capture these frequency patterns and feed them into the device. The device modulates them and returns them via output electrodes to the patient as therapy impulses and the patient and the device form a cybernetic loop.

In practice various effective key settings of the device have emerged for certain disease patterns. These have been listed as therapy programs in the user manual and can be accessed in the Bicom device with a certain number. These empirically identified therapy programs can be used for the majority of patients.

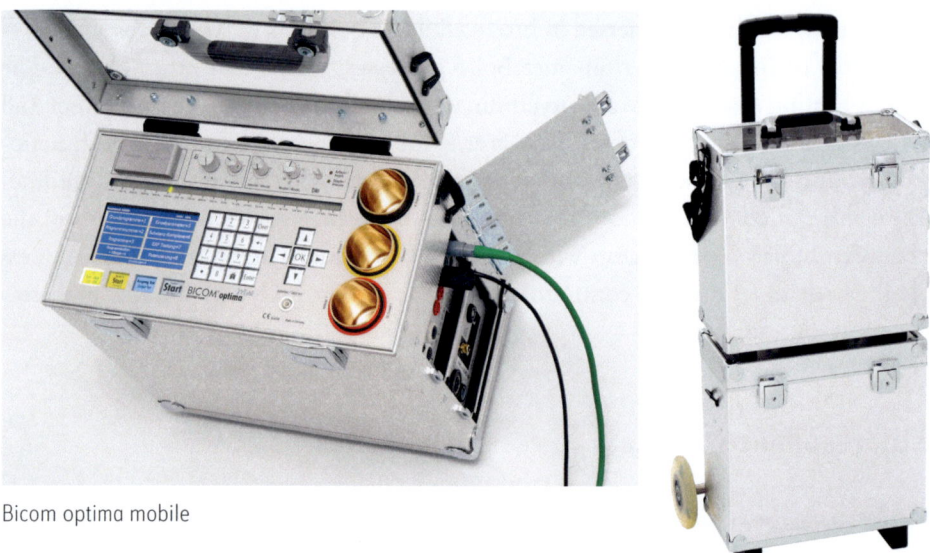

Bicom optima mobile

However, in special cases, the therapist can also select and combine single therapy parameters according to certain rules and perceptions gained in practice and adjust them to the specific patient in order to create an individual therapy program.

Please note that the therapist has to comply with certain basic rules for this procedure. The device itself will not make a diagnosis.

In therapy, the full frequency spectrum available will be used according to the homeopathic simile principle in order to provoke a reaction or divert toxins, for example. The entire inverted, i.e. laterally reversed frequency spectrum will be used to create an energetic balance or divert a toxin or treat an allergy.

A small range within the available frequency spectrum which is defined by the centre frequency (band pass) will be used if only one particular organ or function area is to be addressed. In addition these frequency spectrums can be increased or levelled off. The increase can be applied constantly or it can be increased or levelled off gradually or continuously.

The Bicom device contains an organic filter which is able to separate the patient's frequency spectrum into physiological and pathological frequencies. This allows further interesting combinations of parameters.

Therapy settings which only return the physiological elements to patients are used for exhausted patients or those who are in a bad energetic situation. They will hence be returned their own physiological frequency patterns in a reinforced form in order to strengthen or harmonize them.

The pathological elements of the frequency pattern, which are only applied in inverted form, are mostly used in order to remove interfering fields and in the case of highly acute diseases.

Incidentally there are only very few devices that are able to offer this separation of frequencies and this sophisticated circuit.

The frequency range of the Bicom device is fixed between 1 Hz and 150 kHz. This is the range which is most effective for bioresonance therapy. Higher ranges are less effective for the treatment of diseases. Furthermore long wave frequency ranges and other radio wave frequencies begin beyond 150 kHz.

In addition to the setting described above which is applied though the main therapy channel, the Bicom device provides a second channel which allows information from natural medicine and other stabilizing substances to be applied in parallel to ongoing therapy or in a separate step. This reduces the duration of the therapy. The therapy system presented here offers the opportunity to choose the most suitable frequency pattern from 400 substance complexes.

A further module enables the therapist to apply the Schumann frequencies which have an important function for the well-being of human beings and animals. As these frequencies are often impeded by buildings, asphalt road surfaces and contamination, creatures suffer a deficit that may lead to physical dysfunction.

Using bioresonance with animals

You will, no doubt, ask yourself how all this works in practice – capture oscillation patterns of the patient – modulate them in the device and return them in modulated form to the patient…

To transfer information from the animal to the Bicom device, i.e. the so-called incoming information, we use flexible electrodes, which are usually located at the animal's main energy centres, i.e. in the neck area. Furthermore there are special tapping electrodes for certain applications, for acupuncture, for example, for the treatment of teeth or joints, as well as a magnetic depth probe and various electrodes in special forms like conical, cylindrical or flat electrodes. However, these electrodes are not used solely for inputting information but can also be used for transferring the modulated frequency pattern to the patient, i.e. as output electrodes.

The so-called "modulation mat" is basically used for the outgoing information. This mat is equipped with an additional magnetic field, the intensity of which is less than the earth's magnetic field however. In this context the magnetic field makes the modulated frequency patterns more effective in order to reach right into the body.

These therapeutic frequency patterns can be supported by adding the above-mentioned "dynamic magnetic field impulse"

This magnetic field enables particularly exhausted patients to respond more easily to the applied modulated frequency patterns. This additional magnetic field can be adjusted in terms of intensity and duration – independent of the therapy as such. Furthermore the Bicom optima is able to apply the magnetic field either in a reinforcing or an attenuating form, so that a calming effect is achieved, e.g. with very excited animals or in the case of epileptic animals.

Experience shows the therapeutic effect can even be increased if the therapy cycle is reinforced by adding information from the body's own substances. For this purpose the device has an input electrode in the form of a bowl. It has proven effective to put the following substances into this bowl: faeces in the case of diarrhoea, tear fluid in the case of eye diseases, saliva in the case of diseases of the mouth, blood or hair in the case of skin diseases or – in most cases – blood simply as a general additional information input.

Therapy information occurring during the therapy should be transferred to media which are suitable for storing oscillations. A popular method is to transfer information to a small metal chip which can then be attached to the collar or the halter. An alternative in this context is to place the metal chip in the dog's water bowl. However, this bowl must not be made of metal but preferably of a ceramic material. Another possibility is to store the information in a mixture of water and alcohol. This allows the patient to take the therapeutic information between the usual weekly therapy intervals and to hence extend the therapeutic effect.

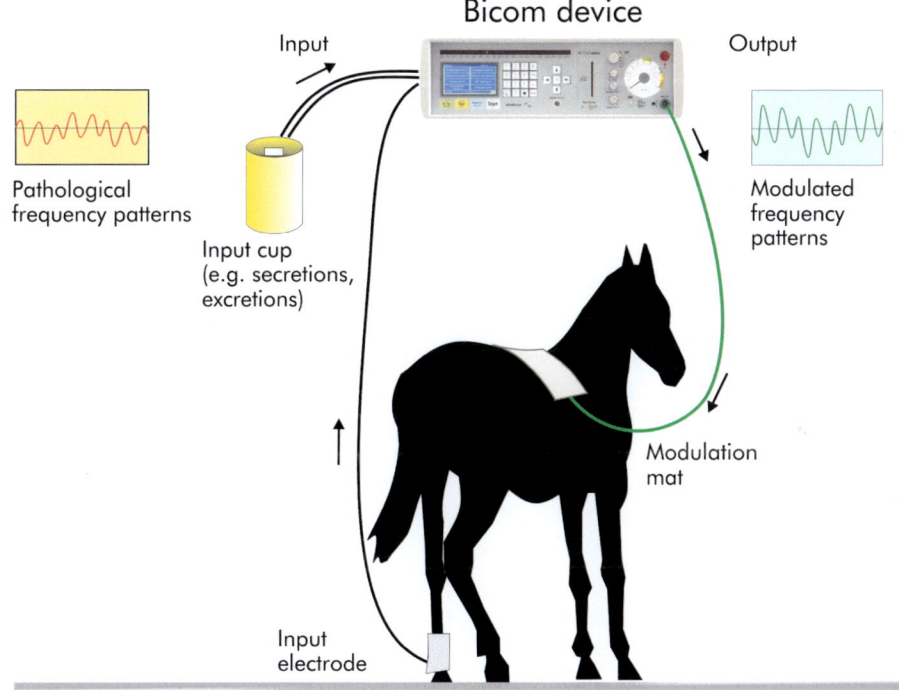

Scheme for applying electrodes to a horse.

The usual course of therapy provides a combination of different programs during which a logical sequence should be observed.

First and foremost in all diseases is therapy of the energetic basic situation. Afterwards the energetic blocks are treated followed by therapy of the eliminating organs in energetic deficit. Finally the energetically disturbed meridians are treated. In the case of infections, toxic stresses and allergies, the so-called eliminating ampullae can be used.

The device provides the opportunity to schedule up to six programs as a proper therapy sequence.

Using the tensor as a biophysical test method

Bioresonance is based on the fact that special frequency patterns go in line with the organism. Information from patients is transferred to the device and is modulated in the device according to the indication. As already explained in the previous chapter, there is a range of possibilities to modulate the input frequency patterns as, for example, through the type of therapy, the amplification and the duration as well as by the choice of frequency.

A total of more than 1,000 different programs are stored in the Bicom optima device. In all those cases where therapy with the chosen programs has limited success, it is the therapist's duty to identify suitable programs for this specific case with the help of energetic tests. In contrast to human medicine, where Voll's electroacupuncture method can be used as a test method due to the measurable skin resistance, we have to apply a different technique in animal medicine because of the coat. In this case, we have to work with a tensor, with a kinesiological method or with pulse testing with RAC according to Nogier.

While kinesiological methods always require a surrogate person and pulse testing is rather impractical because taking the pulse and adjusting the device at the same time is quite difficult, the tensor test is a simple and practicable method to obtain a very good result.

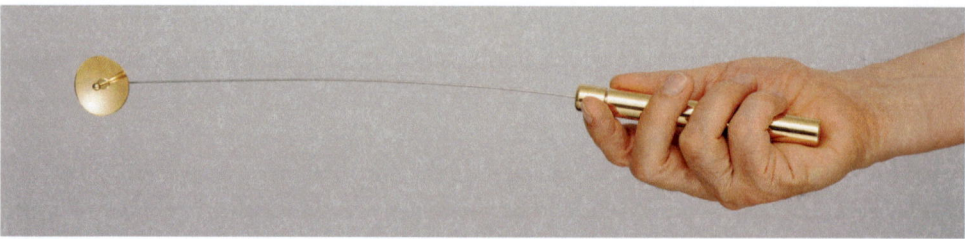

Bio tensor

The term "tensor" refers to a device used for testing electromagnetic oscillation. The tensor consists of a handle, a radial arm and a tensor element. There are various forms of tensor element and the sizes and weights of the various tensors differ considerably. Each therapist must find out which tensor they can work best with. It is advantageous if the tensor can be connected to the device or to a test electrode via a cable.

The tensor is used to check whether the parameters set at the device correspond to the patient. A drop of blood on a filter paper can also be used instead of the actual patient. A simple method is to hold the tensor between an outgoing electrode (modulation mat) and the patient. If both are in line, the tensor will connect the systems by swinging horizontally. In the case of dissonance it will separate the systems by moving up and down.

The tensor technique hence allows us to determine which therapy programs will have a positive effect on the patient or which problem is bothering them and needs to be treated.

Therapy with bioresonance is a relaxing way to be treated.

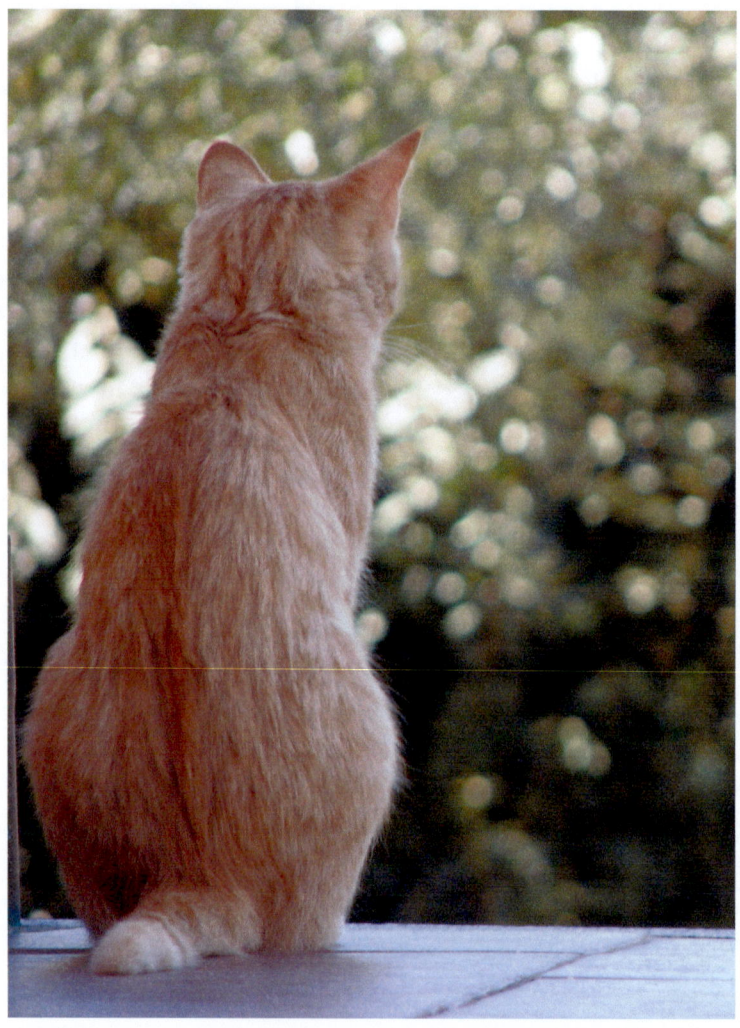

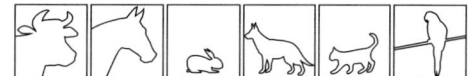

Possibilities of therapy with bioresonance

Healing diseases and helping animals – this is certainly the aim of all students of veterinary medicine. But what happens when they qualify? In most cases practice shows that we tend to look at the symptoms and suppress them, without knowing the cause of the disease however. Suppressing symptoms appears eventually to be successful to a certain extent as the patients are symptom-free. However in many cases other diseases appear in other parts of the organism or similar diseases recur time and time again. Our aim must be to achieve effective healing but in order to reach this aim we must find and eliminate the cause of the disease.

Acute diseases

Using bioresonance in the case of acute diseases? When you read this chapter you might ask yourself whether this does not take too long. Not at all! Anyone who has ever seen a coughing dog entering the practice of a therapist working with bioresonance might find that, after therapy, the cough has gone and the lymph nodes are back to their normal size half a day later when they had been twice this size before. And having seen that, you might recall the numerous cases in conventional medicine where therapy with allopathic medicine required at least three days to produce relief. The cough however remained a lot longer and final recovery took more than one week. The following chapters will show that there is a different way of working.

1. Infectious diseases

In veterinary medicine all diseases transmitted by pathogens are called infectious diseases. The distinction between the various pathogens is done later on, i.e. viruses, germs, fungi and parasites. Contact with the pathogen will occur more often than a manifest and visible disease. However, in veterinary medicine, we mostly see solely those diseased animals. A much larger group of animals will however be able to resist the pathogen when it occurs due to their healthy immune systems and will not show any symptoms.

Daily routine in a vet practice: all the horses in one of the stables are coughing; 30 dogs have come in since last week with loose stools and diarrhoea and a number of cats living in one neighbourhood are suffering from coughs and sneezes. But what about the other animals in that area or, even more surprising, what about the other animals of the same age and breed in the same household that did not fall ill? Mostly we simply tend to say that the immune system of those animals that did not get sick must have been in touch with the pathogen at an earlier stage and is therefore able to resist. But what about the animals of the same age that have always been living in a house or a stable – without any chance of making contact with those pathogens?

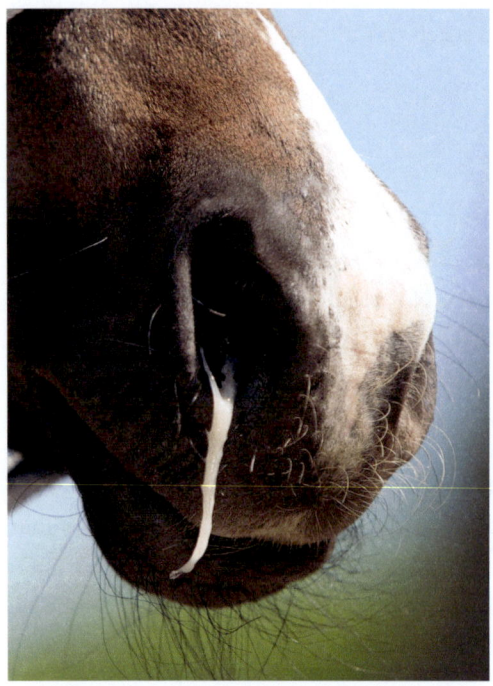

An acute cough and runny nose can be cured quickly with bioresonance therapy.

Let's try to consider how the symptoms of an infectious disease develop and what enables them to devitalize the organism. Don't worry – I will not start to describe the whole biochemical and biophysical route of an agent leading to its pathological symptoms. After all, it can be described in a very simple way: a pathogen makes contact with a host. If the pathogen and the cells of the host are in resonance, disease will break out. If the pathogen does not find any resonance, it will not be able to cause a disease.

The severity of a disease will then depend on the health of the immune system. The organism's immunologically significant mechanisms will do all they can to destroy the invading pathogens and to cure the patient. But very often this will fail at the first attempt because the immune system might be busy with other tasks and is not fully efficient or because a previous infection has prevented the immune system from returning to its full strength.

The rapid success of bioresonance therapy in acute infectious diseases is achieved by bringing the immune system to its full capability and depriving the pathogen of its basic survival needs by inverting its specific oscillation patterns. In my practice I use the Bicom optima which, in the case of viral diseases, allows me to separate the physiological oscillation patterns from the pathological patterns of the virus. It is thus possible to strengthen the physiological parts that are important for the immune system and to invert the weakening oscillation patterns of the virus and hence render the virus harmless to the body. Bioresonance thus enables us to work directly antivirally while conventional medicine is only able to suppress the attending secondary bacterial infections that often occur with antibiotics.

As finally fungi and parasites also have a specific oscillation pattern, we can also restore the patient's health by applying the inverted oscillation patterns as described above with bacterial infections. The aim in the fight against infectious diseases must also be to support the self-healing powers of the body instead of suppressing the symptoms caused by the pathogen. Merely suppressing symptoms will possibly lead to chronic diseases caused by residual agents or even simply by residual information from agents.

2. Sports injuries

Sports injuries with animals – how and when can that happen? While equestrian sports have made up a large part of the spectrum in vet practices for many years now, canine sports have become more important for quite some time too. Looking at slow-motion videos of movement in different animal sports, you become aware of how much the whole musculoskeletal system is affected. Just try to visualize which forces are affecting the foreleg of a horse when it lands after taking a jump. The whole body mass of some 600 kg will compact on this leg. Or think of a dog jumping a hurdle or jumping for a frisbee and landing after a turn in the air.

Or simply imagine yourself jumping from a height of 3 metres, landing on your fingers and pushing back up again right away.

No wonder that pulled tendons or ligaments, spinal problems and sprains of joints and capsules happen time and time again in canine and equine sports. And now go ahead and read the package instructions for the compounds used in conventional medicine: against inflammation, against swelling, against pain – but nothing for improving the tendons, nothing for regenerating the capsule, nothing for restoring function. The overall effect is always "against" a symptom, not "in favour of" healing. Therapists then say that healing

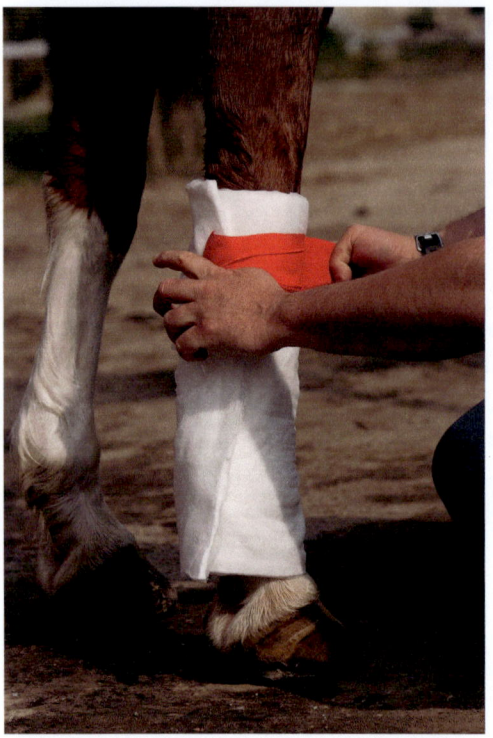

Quick healing without medication is also required in competitive sports.

comes with the necessary rest. But is the tendon able to grow lengthwise allowing normal function and can a capsule grow together without bony growth at the fracture lines and hence a painful arthritic process in the long run all just with the help of rest and controlled movement?

Using bioresonance in sports injuries

This is where the bioresonance method and also the magnetic field should be applied. It doesn't take much imagination to see that again the oscillation pattern of a normal tendon is disturbed after an injury and that it has to be restored. The necessary supporting energy and help to align the single fibres lengthwise is provided by the modulation mat which supplies a magnetic field via the Bicom optima. This leads to significantly quicker healing and avoids subsequent effects that often occur in sports injuries that are treated conventionally. In the case of acute injuries, we place the modulation mat with the healing frequency patterns for this specific injury directly onto the injured part of the body.

In other cases such as general toxin elimination and activation of the lymphatic system as well as the basic program, the mat stays on the back of the animal and the input is also in the area of the main energy zones. The big advantage of the Bicom optima in the case of acute diseases like this is the use of pre-determined frequency patterns allowing the therapist to start the treatment immediately after the clinical diagnosis.

But obvious injuries with significantly impaired movement are not the only areas where bioresonance therapy is effective. Small hidden lesions in the short tendons of the back,

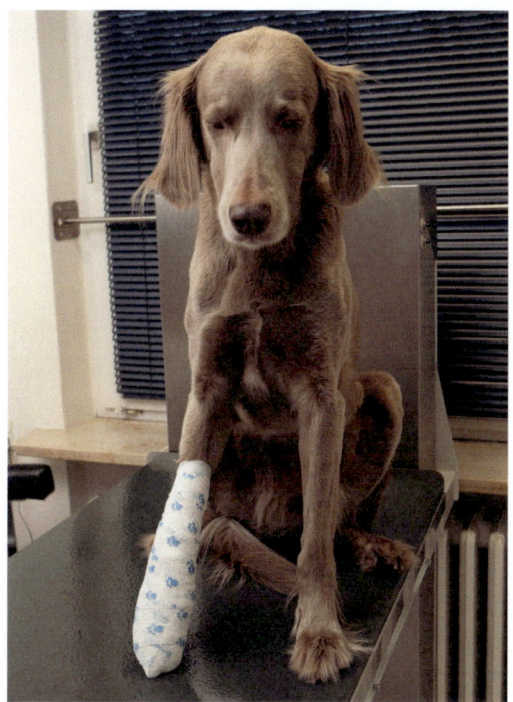

The healing process of a sports injury is shorter with bioresonance therapy and, what is even more important, the dysfunction which often occurs in the course of these diseases can be avoided with bioresonance therapy.

subclinical meniscus problems not yet visible, slightly torn muscle fibres and ligaments – these can also all be energetically detected and healed quickly and efficiently, before more serious damage occurs. Maintenance and monitoring with the Bicom optima can be the key to success in a practice with many patients active in sports and it can cover a large field in a holistic practice.

3. Wound healing

In veterinary medicine we often see infected wounds that won't heal. Bacteria, dirt and permanent licking of the wounds by the patients impede the healing process. Furthermore the tendency, especially in horses, to develop extensive proud flesh is a common complication in the healing of wounds. The bioresonance method can be used in both cases. As we are able to also transfer information to a suitable storage medium, antibacterial programs as well as programs with oscillation patterns for wound healing can be transferred to a special mineral remedy which can be applied locally to the wound, in addition to therapy with the modulation mat on those days between the therapies. Furthermore we can contribute significantly to uncomplicated healing by increasing the body's defences.

4. Chronic diseases

Particularly in the case of chronic diseases of every kind, conventional medicine solely depends upon suppressive therapy which leads to a constantly increasing number of symptoms over the years. The bioresonance method, however, offers the chance to relieve the body of the factors which trigger disease and thus to bring healing. Furthermore, the bioresonance method does not cause any adverse reactions and is free from any nasty accessory symptoms.

a. Allergies

Everybody knows the scenario, be it in the practice or even with our own animals. The dog scratches permanently and everything you have tried was in vain.

Change of food, flea parasiticides, anti-allergic shampoo – no matter what you try, after an initial improvement the situation changes for the worse at the latest after one week. And what is even worse – the longer the trouble lasts, the more problems come along.

Eventually the owner goes to see the vet. We take blood samples, maybe we do a biopsy but whatever effort we make, we don't reach a clear result and hence nor do we achieve a lasting success. The diagnosis usually made would be "complex of allergic problems". Allergic to what? Food? Dust mites? Pollen? Vermin bites? With conventional medicine it is not really possible to find the responsible allergens, other than with very extensive additional examinations.

Food intolerances in dogs have been constantly increasing throughout recent years. But which food can the dog cope with? The usual advice is to put it on a so-called exclusion diet. A common suggestion would be horse meat with potatoes since most dogs have not yet been in contact with those two components during their life. But if the dog still continues scratching, it might also be allergic to an environmental factor such as dust mites or pollen, especially in summer. It was not until I started working with bioresonance that I was finally able to achieve a breakthrough in treating allergies in my practice.

An allergy is a disorder of the immune system. Bioresonance aims to eliminate this disorder and to put the immune reactions in disorder back on the right track.

Bioresonance works with specific frequency patterns of the body's electromagnetic field and of the pathological substances. It has an influence on the control processes, e.g. also on the immune system.

With the help of these specific frequency patterns, we can test allergens but also pathogenic environmental toxins, fungi, viruses, bacteria etc.

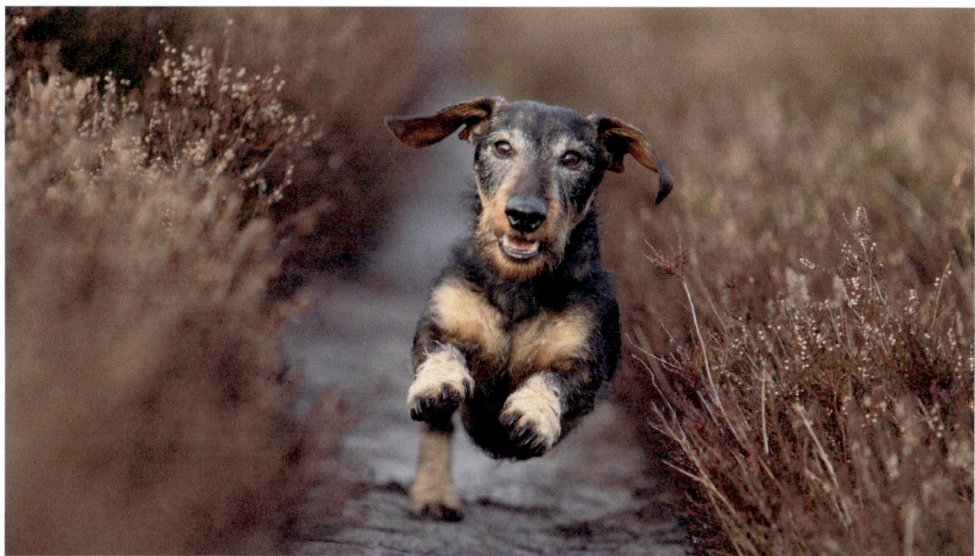

Only a dog that is free from allergies can show so much lust for life.

If you know the cause of an allergic reaction in the body, the easiest way to ease the pain of the animal would be to keep it away from the trigger. Unfortunately this is not always possible and in many cases it isn't enough either. On the one hand, allergies often accumulate in the body over a prolonged period of time and more and more allergens come along. On the other hand, simply avoiding the allergen is, in many cases, impossible. For instance, what do you do if a dog reacts to all proteins in various types of meat? This is something that happens increasingly often. The same goes if an allergy to dust mites is diagnosed - this is a real problem for the dog because how can you avoid dust?

Detoxification with bioresonance

Fortunately bioresonance is not only a great system for diagnosing patients but also a fantastic form of therapy . And, in therapy, the focus is once again not only on treating the symptom, e.g. the itching, but on getting to the root of the problem and systematically fighting the cause allowing the body to react normally again.

With the help of bioresonance we are able to eliminate the harmful substance from the organism.

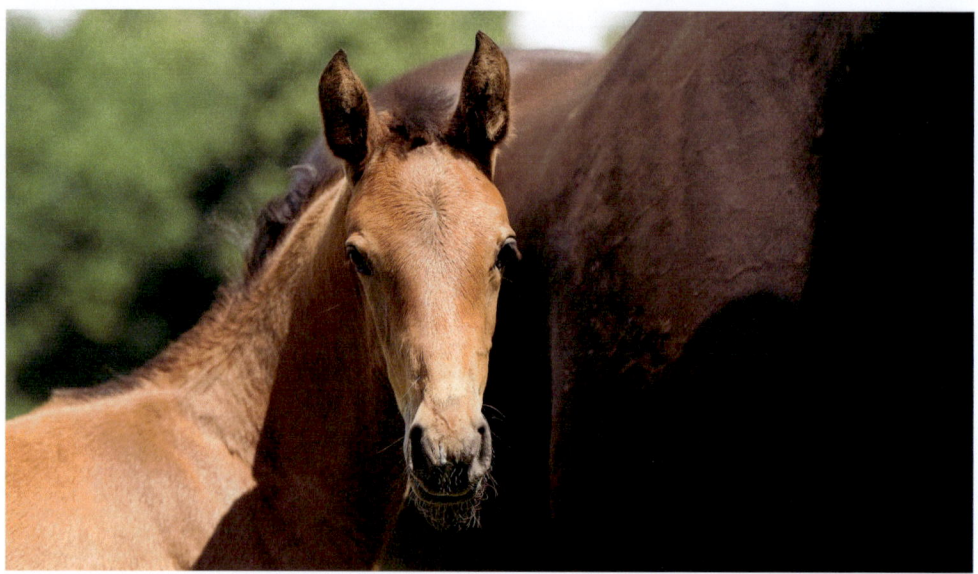

During the developmental stage of young animals, in particular, we must attach great importance to a healthy upbringing in order to avoid long-term damage.

Just think of mercury or aluminium particles contained in injection compounds, car emissions our dogs are exposed to due to their height, synthetic particles released by food and water bowls, food that is contaminated with toxins or think of bacterial or viral infections that have not been fully cured or that occurred only subliminally. And, finally, stress can also have a negative effect on the body's self-regulation.

In all cases of chronic disease we must not forget that some of our animals carry massive energetic blocks in their bodies, some of which are significant due to a large amount of accumulated toxins. Therefore each and every bioresonance therapy must always begin by testing blocks in the organism and treating them. Sometimes these tests show very surprising results.

For instance I was presented a brood bitch that did not have a regular heat cycle for almost 2 years and did not get pregnant. Conventional examinations were unable to provide a diagnosis. But when the biophysical test showed that, among other problems, the bitch was suffering from radiation exposure, we found that she was sleeping close to the wireless LAN and next to the computer. After her basket was moved and she was treated three times with bioresonance she immediately came into heat, was mated and later on gave birth to 8 healthy pups.

A further case of a dog that was sick due to blocks was one that was suffering from massive allergies where I found geopathic[1] stress. As the dog was living in the German area called the "Volcanic Eifel", we were not able to change the geological situation responsible for the geopathic stress but the owners of the dog were willing for a geopathologist to suppress their house and the dog's geopathic stress was then treated successfully with bioresonance. The allergy itself was then removed easily with further allergy programs during bioresonance therapy.

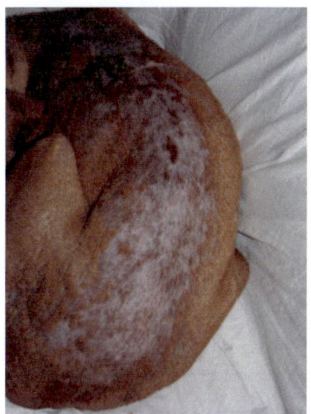 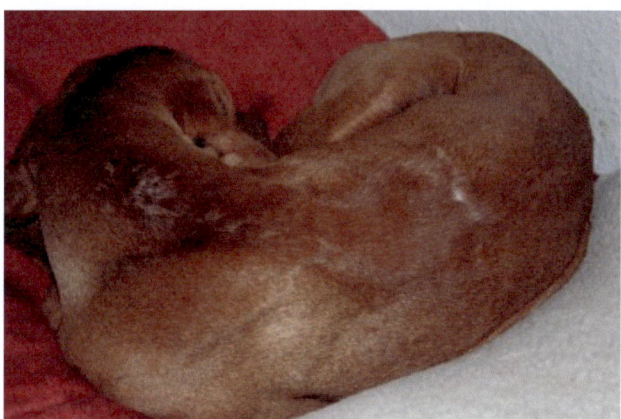

Bioresonance therapy can lead to visible healing after just three treatments.

In most cases of allergies the functioning of one or more eliminating organs is in disorder which leads to the problem that toxins are not sufficiently excreted. These organ systems must also be supported by bioresonance therapy.

The problems of an allergic animal mostly appear at the following main excretory organs:

Skin   – the skin modifies or itches and we often see recurring otitis
Bowel – pasty defecations
Lung   – asthma-like symptoms, chronic bronchitis

In the case of horses, in particular, we must clearly consider those with chronic bronchitis as allergic. In these cases it is essential to clarify whether there is contamination with fungi as most horses suffering from COPD show mould fungi as their main problem.

---

[1]   Geopathy: energetic stress caused by the earth interfering (e.g. watercourses, fault lines etc)

However, ultimately, we have to acknowledge that the symptoms of the allergic animal only show the outward indication of an inner dysregulation.

As bioresonance starts at the control level and aims to remedy the dysfunction of the immune system, it is possible to heal the allergy with bioresonance. If possible, a certain period away from exposure to the allergen is also helpful in bioresonance therapy. However, even if this is not feasible, therapy is still possible. I remember a case of a terrier living together with two cats that was allergic to the cats' hair. After bioresonance therapy he was able to live happily with his four-legged friends without any allergic symptoms.

Following successful therapy with bioresonance, the organism is able to recognize those substances which it used to consider as allergens as no longer harmful and will no longer show any allergic reaction.

b. When metabolism is at sixes and sevens

We hear it time and time again in the practice – my dog is drinking enormous amounts of water, my tomcat is losing his hair, my horse has problems changing his coat and his performance drops during the summer.

What is behind animal owners tell us something like this? In many cases clinical examinations of the mucosa, the lungs, the heart and the abdominal organs don't reveal any results. Sometimes the owners report vomiting or diarrhoea or alternating soft stools.

These hints can lead us to presume an organic disease of the kidneys, but it may also be diabetes mellitus, commonly called diabetes.

In order to confirm the suspected diagnosis or to exclude this disease we first have to do a clinical blood count including all relevant serum levels.

Once the diagnosis kidney failure or diabetes has been confirmed, what are you going to do? According to conventional medicine neither disease can be cured but can only be treated to a certain extent in the long term and the duration of therapy is limited due to the massive complications and side-effects. Furthermore, in most cases, the owner of the patient must be able to inject his own animal and stick to a very detailed injection and nutrition schedule.

In the case of kidney failure the situation is often even worse because classic conventional medicine offers no treatment beyond dietary measures or blood pressure compounds in order to lower the blood pressure in the stressed vessels.

But let us leave these two common diseases in dogs and cats and have a look at other diseases that also occur with vomiting and alternating stools.

One disease that belongs to this complex of symptoms is so-called hepatic inflammation or hepatitis. However it must not be confused with hepatitis I to III in humans. Hepatitis in animals is an inflammatory reaction of the liver cells with resulting dysfunction of the liver

Again classic conventional medicine cannot do much more than merely protect, although real protective therapy of the liver does not exist. Eventually conventional medicine can only relieve the liver with a specific diet and can furthermore add supplements to deliver amino acids and vitamins that are necessary for effective metabolism of the liver. In this case the owner of the animal can only hope that the liver is able to recover with the help of the liver diet.

Of course diseases of the liver do not only appear in dogs, cats and small animals. Large animals and here in particular, cattle and horses, suffer quite often from liver disease which is a considerable problem in view of the increased performance requirements. This goes for performance in equestrian sports as well as milk and fattening performance in cattle. And these diseases often lead to a decline in performance e.g. in the middle of the show season in equestrian sports. Likewise a delayed change of coat or extensive loss of fur in our four-legged friends can often be a symptom of a liver disease.

In the context of a blood count of diseased animals you will, however, often find not only increased serum levels of those data characteristic of liver and kidney function, but also a reduced number of red blood cells and haematocrit value. As the red blood cells are responsible for the smooth transport of oxygen to the tissue, there is hardly any doubt why the animal presented to you feels so bad.

In all these cases, classic conventional medicine is usually unable to explain the cause of the disease. At best conventional medical treatment can support the self-healing process.

One further complex of diseases that so far can only be treated, but not healed, with conventional medicine is Cushing's syndrome. This is a disease where the body's own cortisone level is increased – either due to increased function of the adrenal cortex or due to increased production of stimulating hormones in the brain. The phenomenon is mainly visible through altered growth of the coat. Most dogs will show hairless sports with parchment-like skin while most horses show a much delayed change of coat.

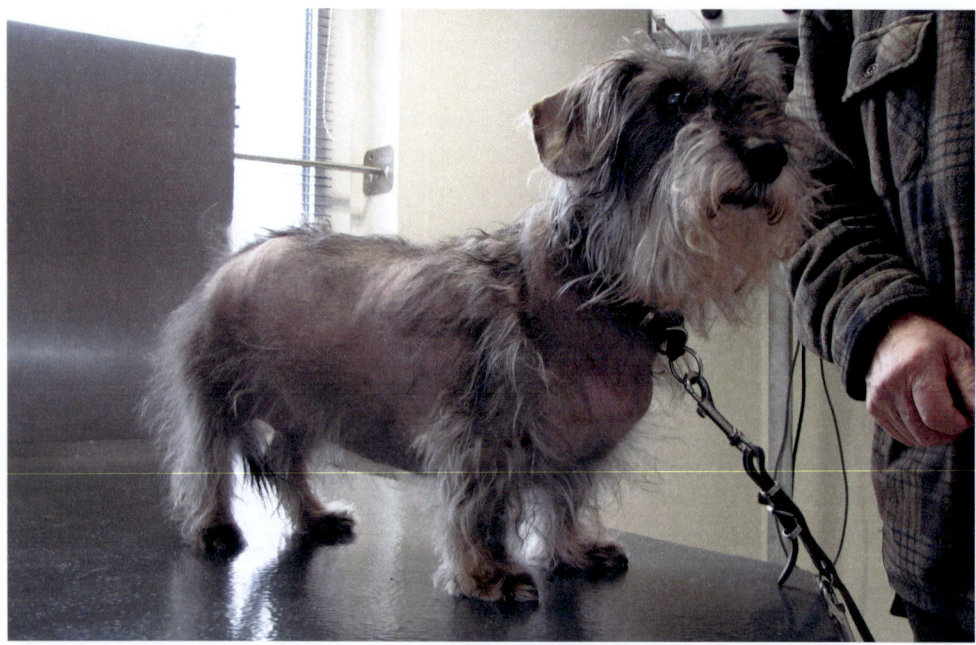

Despite suffering from Cushing's disease for more than two years, this Dachshund was healed with bioresonance.

Now, looking at all these different examples of various metabolic disorders, you will have noted that one crucial question has not been answered: "Why does one individual suffer from this disease while another one does not?" Conventional medicine is only able to diagnose an animal with disease. And this diagnosis cannot be made until it has developed to an extent that measurable parameters exist.

In the context of kidney failure, in particular, the point of time of the diagnosis, however, is very late. Measurable serum values of urea and creatinine will not be noticed in the blood until 75% of both kidneys are in disorder.

However, conventional medicine will not reveal what makes an organism start the deficient development leading to these diseases.

In those cases we use the bioresonance method in our practice. In order to understand the way it works, we have to return once more to the theory of bioresonance.

Bioresonance therapy benefits from the fact that each individual shows a certain oscillation pattern that can be measured using a particular testing procedure.

The specific oscillations or oscillation patterns corresponding to the individual tissue, i.e. also to organs, indicate which specific organ is in disorder through disturbed flow of information between the individual cells.

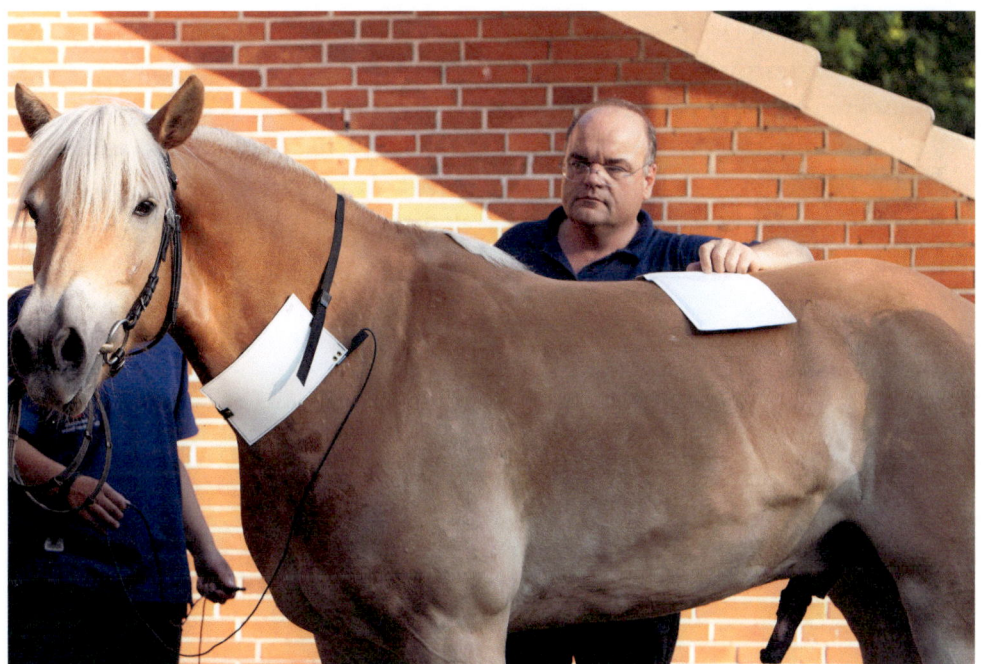

A relaxed horse enjoying treatment with bioresonance.

Bioresonance thus does not consider a single blood value to be diagnosed but the body as a whole. It is essential to find out which of the individual's organs are disturbed and, most of all, which problem affecting the organism has led to this dysfunction.

Once we have found the disturbing cause, we will be able to treat the body with the corresponding bioresonance oscillations (oscillation patterns) so that the organism is relieved from this problem and the organs can recommence their normal function.

The test will identify the type of individual problem - whether it is viral, bacterial, parasitic or metallic. Possible dysfunction of organs due to stress will also be visible.

Any organic disease, or rather any organic disease diagnosed with conventional medicine, will first require determination of the basic energetic situation of the organism. After all only an organism that is able to react or that has been re-enabled with the help of bioresonance to react can deal with its problems.

The subsequent bio-energetic examination which must not be neglected will then deal with the energetic blocks[2] that cause the individual problems. Among those problems are blocks of the spine in horses doing equestrian sports, for example. These blocks may cause problems in the horse's rideability. But likewise other blocks such as scars, dysfunctions of the acid-base-balance, vaccination blocks, geopathic problems, and blocks in the temporomandibular joint or in the lingual bone, all these blocks may contribute considerably to the development of organic problems. But all these blocks can be detected and, more importantly, treated with the help of bioresonance analysis.

Only further examination of the so-called eliminating organs with the help of the pre-stored program parameters will reveal which organ and its function are significantly stressing the body.

As the bioresonance test works directly with the relevant therapy frequencies, nothing prevents the treatment's positive influence on energetic dysfunction and hence the complete recovery of functioning.

---

[2] energetic block: a factor preventing the energy in the body from flowing normally

In conventional medicine, dysfunctions of the metabolic system cannot be treated at all or only by permanently prescribing medication. The aim of therapy must therefore be to find the real cause of the disease instead of suppressing the symptoms and to finally re-establish a working and healthy physiological system in the animal.

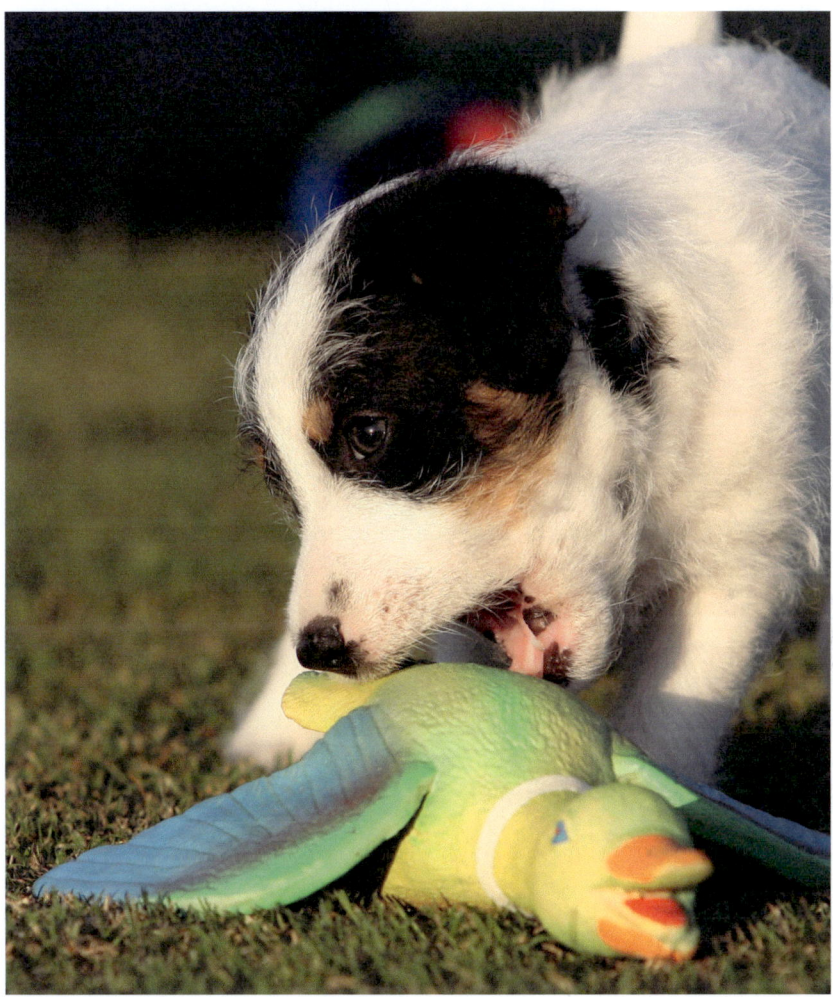

Bioresonance has helped this happy little pup.

c. Gastro-intestinal diseases

Constantly recurring colic with horses, so-called stool water, poor performance due to abdominal cramps, recurring diarrhoea with dogs, soft stools and/or stools covered with mucus, frequent vomiting with cats and dogs – all these problems are things you see every day in your vet practice. And without bioresonance you are restricted to treating most of them merely with symptomatic therapies and diets

Many is the time that I have seen people in the practice start flapping just because we asked them whether we were allowed to give their dog a treat and who told us that even the smallest crumb of different food would cause bloody diarrhoea. What a fiasco – at least this is what I am thinking since I have introduced bioresonance in my practice. The poor dog is not allowed any treats and never eats anything but the "special intestinal diet food" by So-and-so or whatever all these so-called "extra healthy" dog foods are called. And ultimately all this special food has one aim: please don't stress the intestines with any substance that might get the intestinal mucosa working. But it is so simple - take the information of the diseased intestines (e.g. put stools in the input bowl), have the pathological frequency pattern modulated by the device and return the modulated oscillation pattern to the dog. In many cases the intestinal mucosa will regenerate. And the same effect will be found in horses and other animals. In the case of intestinal disorders we modulate the pathological oscillation and use the resulting modulated information to restore the animal's health.

But it isn't always that easy. What is the cause of this digestive disorder? Is it a pathologically altered intestinal wall in which the intestinal cells secrete water instead of absorbing it? Is the intestinal environment in disorder? Is there an infestation with Candida? Is it an allergy to certain foods? Wheat? Milk? Eggs?

You will certainly say that your dog does not get any milk and your horse even less. But can you be sure that your dog food does not contain any trace of milk power as a source of protein? Does the declaration on the feedbag really show us the true content? Probably not...

There are limits that have to be exceeded before one or other ingredient has to be stated on the declaration. Apart from that, each foodstuff may contain contamination by third parties – for instance with substances that the cereals contained in the food have absorbed while growing in the field. Or they might be contaminated with substances from those animals utilized in the production of this food and which those animals might have acquired due to their upkeep or their food. In this context I would like to mention a warning notice from the German Federal Government published in the year 2010 in which they strongly recommended avoiding overeating sunflower seeds because of increased content of cadmium as well as the intensive consumption of tuna due to the high content of mercury and finally the regular consumption of cod liver oil due to the high content of polychlorinated biphenyls (PCBs - c.f. dioxin).

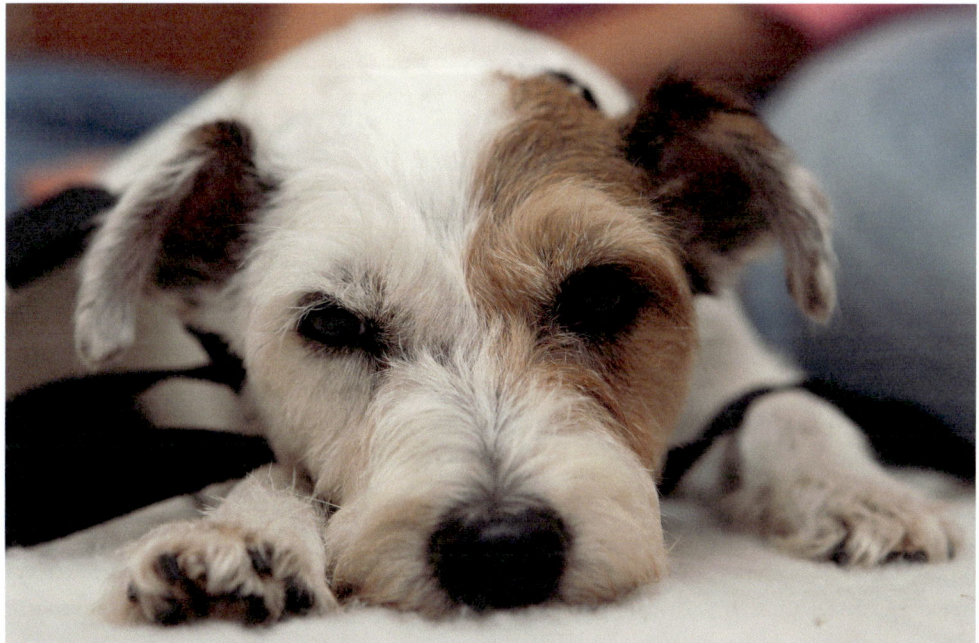

A relaxed dog enjoying bioresonance therapy.

In conventional medicine all these various possibilities cannot really be diagnosed. However, with the bioresonance method and its biophysical diagnostic methods, diagnosis is quite simple. And once you know the enemy you are fighting against, healing is as easy as anything. For most substances there are "reference ampoules"[3] that contain the information stored in energetic form. The decisive step is therapy with the assistance of known

---

[3] Reference ampoules: these ampoules contain the specific information of a substance stored on a fluid and they can be used for testing in the surrounding area

pathological oscillation patterns and their modulation. Of course you should consider microbiological intestinal rehabilitation in case the intestinal environment is in disorder. Detoxification of Candida together with rehabilitation of the intestinal flora with the intestinal bacteria specific to the particular animal will then lead to healthy intestines.

Every vet specialized in the treatment of small animals knows the problems with diets in animals and their acceptance by owners and animals. In some cases the bioresonance method may have to be supported by a diet; however, this is usually only necessary for around 4 weeks and should thus be acceptable for every owner.

The restoration of a normal gastro-intestinal system and a healthy intestinal environment plays a decisive role in all immunological diseases. Nearly all immunological settings in the organism take place in the intestines. In terms of anatomy, the main contribution to a healthy immune system is provided by an agglomeration of numerous lymph nodes called "Peyer's plaques". After all there is a reason why the development of all kinds of allergies is always related to a disturbed immune system and disturbed intestinal flora.

d. Diseases of the urological complex

You may know the situation: cystitis recurs time and time again, antibiotics are given one by one and, if you are lucky, the chronic inflammation of the bladder will heal despite the permanent administration of antibiotics. This would be a mischievous, but sadly true, description because, in the long run, the cause of this painful and persistent chronic cystitis is not so much the bacteria. The disturbed immune system and a susceptible bladder mucosa certainly are factors that are much more likely to be the cause. Fighting the bacteria hence is a measure that is only effective on the surface of the disease. We must therefore aim at changing the body's defence so that a bacterial attack does not stand a chance. In general recurrent cystitis is definitely a chronic disease and the main task is to find the cause and eliminate it. As already described in the previous chapter, disturbed intestinal immunity can also be a reason for a disturbed defence system. After having tested the negative factors that are causing the disease and after treating them, pathological alteration of the bladder mucosa is only a small further step in the therapy.

Here, again, the holistic view of a disease plays the lead. Each therapy with bioresonance should always begin with the basic energetic situation with regard to the organism's ability to regulate itself. In these diseases, too, the next step is to determine the blocks preventing the body from healing itself. The next step is to improve the function of the deficient eliminating organs with a subsequent program chain adapted to the specific indications. Finally the organism is stabilized with the help of the meridian programs[4]. The elimination of specific stresses, be they bacterial, viral, metallic or any other kind, must therefore be integrated as a necessary step in the overall therapy concept.

However the urological field does not just cover recurrent cystitis but – mainly in cats – the treatment of crystalline deposits, also called urinary gravel or, in the case of large crystals, urinary stones. Let's visualize how such flocculation is caused.

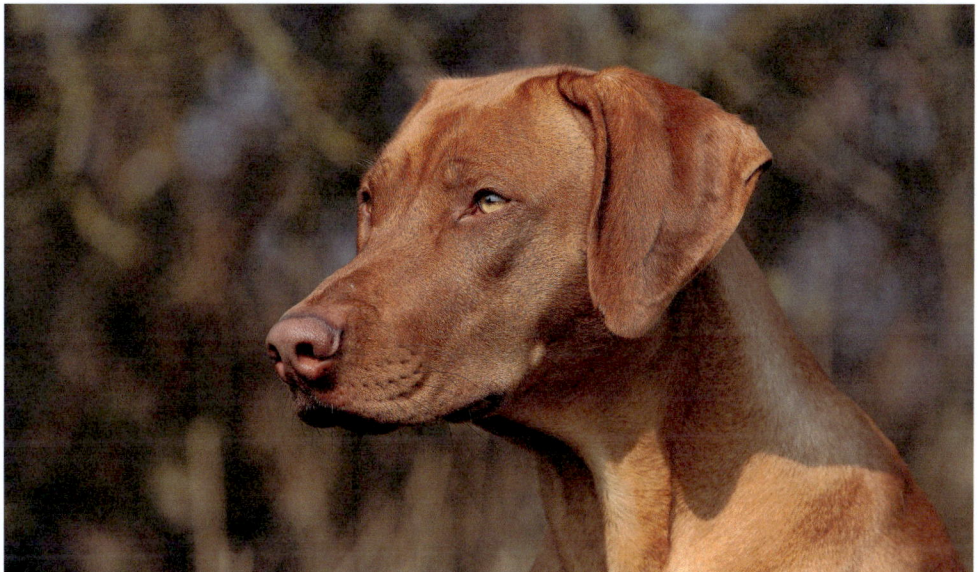

A healthy dog with a keen expression.

Development of flocculation

Urine is a liquid that consists of several components and which has a specific acidity (pH value) in each animal species. If one of these components is in disorder, e.g. if the pH value of a cat is alkaline, the cat will develop crystals, in this case mostly struvite floccu-

---

4   Meridian program: meridians are energy gates which, according to traditional Chinese acupuncture, are crucial for regulation in both human and animal bodies

lation. Conventional medicine is not sure of the reason for the disturbed composition of the urine and calls it a metabolic disorder. However bioresonance offers the possibility to energetically find the reason for the disease and to lay the foundation for restoring normal metabolism. Here, too, we have to find the pathological frequency pattern and return it with the help of the modulation mat supported by the magnetic field. Once again the bioresonance method is the only possibility to recreate a healthy organism. In the end the bioresonance method, just like acupuncture and homeopathy, is a regulative therapy with the aim of encouraging the body's self-healing process and restoring its health.

e. Fertility problems

Bioresonance therapy can also be used in a very effective way to treat fertility problems in our pets and livestock. Many bitches, female cats and horses have been successfully treated with bioresonance helping them to become pregnant.

In this context I remember a 16-year-old mare that did not get pregnant on a stud farm for 2 years despite intensive hormonal treatment. Maybe I should say "because of" hormonal treatment. It was clear that, according to conventional medicine, there was no reason why the mare did not get pregnant and therefore the vets tried everything that chemistry had to offer.

This interpretation certainly is quite sarcastic – mainly against the background that all those ever so great diagnostic methods of conventional medicine were exploited. But the final result is exactly what my experience shows: bioresonance therapy is a successful method even in these apparently hopeless cases.

And it is so easy to comprehend: a pathological oscillation pattern in the organism causes a disorder somewhere in the body. Finding and treating this oscillation pattern in order to restore the physiological oscillation is the aim of bioresonance.

In the case of this mare, the various diagnostic steps in the bioresonance method with Bicom optima were carried out as usual and what I found was: the basic energetic state was blocked in its reaction, a medicine block was in place – not surprising in view of the patient's history – the eliminating organs found were the kidneys and the uterus. In addition I found specific problems in the area of the kidney and liver meridians caused by herpes viruses, Streptococci and Pasteurella as well as Candida infection.

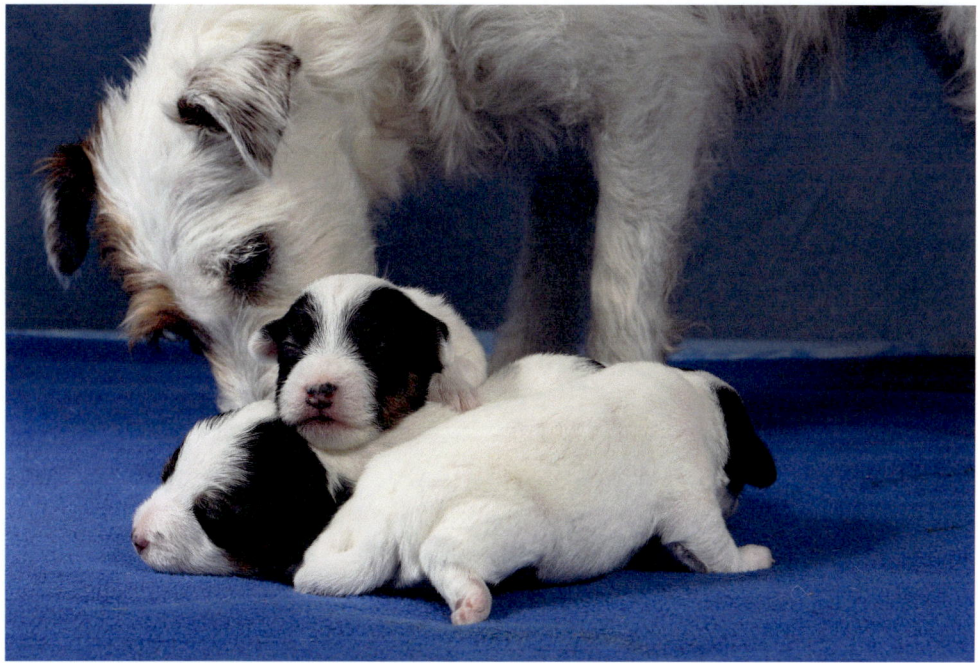

A pretty and healthy litter thanks to bioresonance therapy after the treatment of fertility problems.

Therapeutical approach with the Bicom device

In the case of such an extremely disturbed patient, initial treatments must always concentrate on restoring energetic responsiveness as well as removing the blocks affecting the patient and also stimulating the deficient eliminating organs. Time and again it is amazing to see that even animals that are totally exhausted feel much better already after the first therapy. Many owners report that, already in the first few days following initial treatment, their animals exhibit behaviour they have not seen in a long time – they frolic and romp around, roll over, start cleaning themselves and appear to be much happier.

By the way, it is very important that you, as the therapist, urge the owner of the animal to always provide sufficient fresh water. After all the toxins are losing their ground in the organism and have to be washed out.

After the first three sessions, I always re-test the animals in my practice with the Bicom optima because I want to find which stresses and blocks have already changed or have even disappeared. In some cases it may happen that, after the first treatment, new stresses emerge and can be treated. In the case of the mare described above, this new test revealed an additional infection with Staphylococci that was hidden in the overall situation at the first examination. We subsequently channelled the stresses in a series of six treatments. When we tested the mare again after the final treatment, no further stresses were found. Both the owner and I waited optimistically for the mare to come into season, which she did after one week. The mare was inseminated and her foal is now two years old.

Here's a further case of a bitch to show that this was not an isolated case. For this bitch conventional medicine would have been able to advertise a professorship if only somebody had been successful in breeding from this dog. But neither professional examinations at various renowned clinics nor various attempts at insemination and natural matings brought success. As the bloodlines of this bitch were very valuable for the breed, the breeder did not want to give up on her. Meanwhile the bitch was already 6 years old and it was about time for her first pregnancy.

I examined the bitch with the bioresonance method. The basic program in terms of energetic responsiveness which the animal needed was the program for animals blocked in their reactivity. The block unveiled by the test was a geopathic disorder in terms of exposure to electronic smog and the eliminating organs that were deficient were the kidney and the uterus. Both the kidney and the female sex hormones showed a specific meridian problem. Although I would have expected an additional bacterial or viral stress, the bitch did not show any of these particular stresses and energetic testing showed nothing but abnormal elimination.

Now the most difficult task was to discuss with the animal's owner possible geopathic factors in her environment and to convince her that this was one of the reasons that her bitch did not get pregnant. In the case of geopathic factors, we are able to restore the organism with bioresonance therapy, but further damage to the body can be expected if the geopathic disorder persists. During conversation with the owner she told me that the bitches' favourite place was next to the WLAN device in the hall. Although she was somewhat disbelieving in the beginning, she was prepared to turn the WLAN off at night and to move the animal's sleeping place to a different room.

The bitch was then treated three times against the geopathic disorder at weekly intervals and came into season after just the second treatment. According to her owner this heat was very strong and, on my advice, she was mated. The healthy pups are now also two years old. The bitch has remained healthy and has never exhibited any disorder of her hormonal balance since then.

f. Endocrine disorders

Independent of the hormonal imbalances in relation to infertility already discussed, we are very often also able to intervene with bioresonance in disease complexes such as thyroid dysfunction for example, mostly as a support but also as a healing therapy.

Ultimately, both forms of the disease do not exist directly after birth but in most cases they appear in the adult animal. Again we mainly have to ask for the why and wherefore as the primary basis for our therapy. An organism that was obviously healthy in the beginning suddenly becomes sick. Serological examination of the blood count reveals hypothyrosis. Conventional medicine knows various causes for this disease: auto-antibodies against the thyroid hormone, production of TSH has fallen short, too little conversion in the thyroid. But what was the cause?

Unfortunately conventional medicine cannot provide an explanation. People talk of metabolism problems, too little iodine in the food and other things but all of this does not help to find the cure. What has prevented the body from maintaining normal thyroid function?

Significance of the thyroid

Holistic and natural medicine has been aware for a very long time that the thyroid is extremely active in overall metabolism and is one of the excretory organs. Conventional medicine has found small insignificant nodules in the thyroids that enlarge and get smaller again but do not show any pathological result, even in scintigraphy. These are called "trivial adenomas", without realising that this is exactly the place where elimination is dysfunctional.

Heavy metals, contamination with bacteria, fungi, chemicals or viral stresses and many more are the crucial keywords for processes disturbing the metabolism. Of course, here again, we have to start energetic examination before beginning the therapy. Also, in these cases, the energetic ability to regulate must be restored first. The second step in successfully treating thyroid disease is to search for energetic blocks, interference fields caused by scars, quinsy, geopathic factors, Candida, jaw joint blocks, blocks of the sympathetic chain in the neck and treat these disorders.

Furthermore the Bicom optima provides preinstalled programs that can be tested in the diagnosis of a thyroid problem and they can also be used for therapy. It goes without saying that, when treating a block of the excretory organs, it is essential to support those organs that show an energetic deficit. In most cases markedly improved well-being can already be noted after these basic therapies, sometimes even after just one treatment. However, the aim of therapy must be to avoid prescribing tablets and to achieve the final cure. It is essential to test the individual stresses with a proven diagnostic method, the so-called "combined testing technique" (CTT) and to carry out therapy accordingly.

Ultimately the diagnosed pathological oscillation pattern and its modulated form are crucial for the success of the therapy. After diagnosing and consistently treating as well as eliminating the individual stresses, I am happy to look back at several cases in my practice where follow-up with conventional medicine no longer showed any thyroid disorder, even with the stimulation test. A few other cases were not healed completely but at least we were able to reduce the amount of tablets by half, in some cases even significantly more.

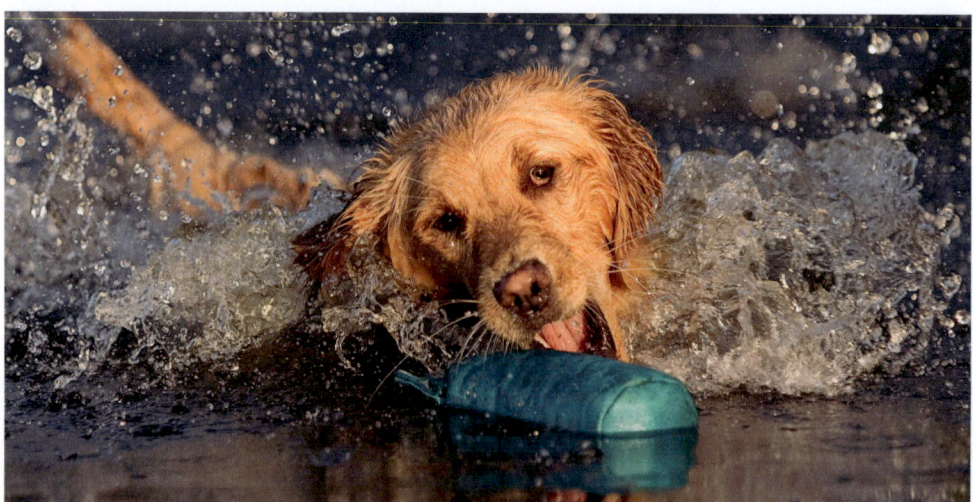

The aim in veterinary medicine with bioresonance is a happy and active animal.

g. Movement disorders – lameness

I have heard it many times in orthopaedics: my horse is lame, my dog doesn't want to move, and my cat walks with a limp. Many complex and expensive examinations are carried out – all without any pathological result. The horse must have twisted its ankle, the dog must have fallen, and the cat just has a distortion. Therapy: general anti-inflammatories, painkillers, bandages on the joints that are assumed to be the location of the pain. Of course it is possible that an animal has sprained its paw but this is a rather rare event. In most cases this vague lameness is caused by disorders of the energy flow and this must be fixed.

Disorders of the energy flow are nothing special for those therapists who have studied acupuncture. They talk about blocks of the spine or about energetic jams in the meridians along the limbs. But which ones?

Diagnosis with the tensor

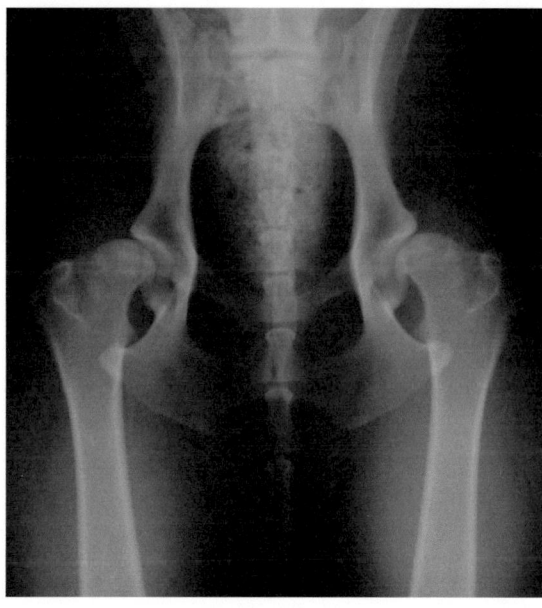

Severe hip arthrosis in a dog.

In this context bioresonance and its examination technique with the tensor makes life much easier. The tensor can be connected easily with the magnetic depth probe[5]. If you now tap the obviously diseased limbs with the magnetic depth probe and the tensor or go along the spine with the magnetic depth probe, you will immediately become aware of where the block is located. In acute cases it will be sufficient to treat this area with the pre-installed programs. The energy flow will immediately be restored and, in most cases, an improvement in the gait can be seen right after the first therapy.

---

[5] Magnetic depth probe: a small instrument with a strong permanent magnetic field that can also be used for testing.

The pre-installed specific and non-specific pain programs are also a blessing in breaking the vicious circle created by the pain and in enabling normal movement again. My patients in serious sports, in particular, have been treated with incredible success and all this without any kind of doping so that bioresonance can even be used during the tournament season.

With chronic patients it sometimes takes a bit longer to succeed but here, too we are very successful even if the X-rays show distinctive alterations. Of course exostosis cannot always be removed but we have seen time and time again in my practice that, even in the case of severe X-ray findings, the bony structures improved or that, after osteolytic processes, healthy bone tissue developed. In principle this is quite easy to explain. As bony reactions are often a result of static alterations, restoration of the normal course of movement will also lead to remission of the bony processes. But of course these diseases

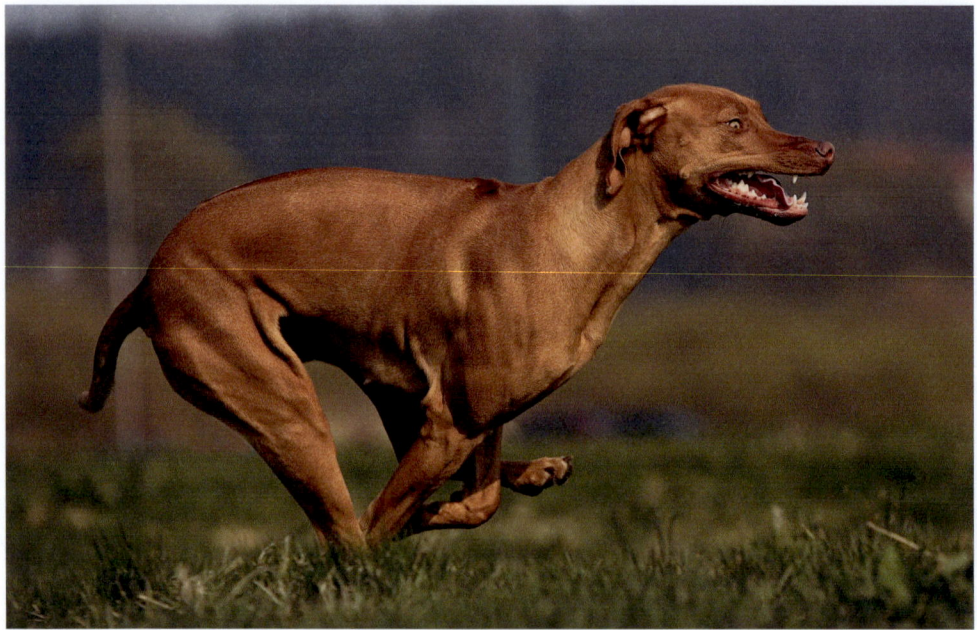

A healthy dog after bioresonance therapy for orthopaedic problems.

also require the usual course of therapy.

Especially in the case of chronic diseases of the musculoskeletal system, we often see stresses from bacterial diseases and here, in particular, infection with Borrelia. Elimination of these stresses with bioresonance and the use of nosodes[6] prepared especially for the particular patient will ultimately lead to success. Therapy with nosodes will be dealt with in a later chapter.

h. Diseases of the spine

A typical case in every vet practice: Mrs. Smith comes with her dachshund as an emergency case. One hour ago Billy jumped from the sofa, whined briefly and now he can hardly move. Billy is no longer able to coordinate his hind legs.

The therapist now has to do the classic course of a neurological examination and, in most cases, the final diagnosis will be "intervertebral disc disease". In conventional medicine this disease describes a dysfunction of the spinal cord. The cause for this disturbed function mostly is a herniated disk that is contusing the nerves in the spinal cord. The disk itself mostly dissolves so that the contusion is caused by a swelling of the nerve sheaths caused by the remains of the vertebral body in the spinal cord.

As Billy is still able to pass urine and stools and as he has not suffered a total loss of sensitivity, the therapists agrees with the owner to treat the little four-legged friend with bioresonance.

Therapy by means of bioresonance

The aim of therapy must be the quick reduction of the swelling allowing the energy flow in the nerves to be restored and to avoid irreversible destruction of the nerves. Billy can be treated quickly and painlessly with the bioresonance programs for toxin elimination and activation of the lymphatic system.

During the first days of the disease, the treatment is carried out every 2 to 3 days and can be changed to a weekly interval after 3 to 4 treatments. Already after the second session Billy walked happily into the practice. The coordination problems in the hind legs were only visible when he moved quickly. After a total of 6 therapies, Billy was back to his old self again and enjoyed life as before.

---

[6] Nosodes: potentiated toxins of all kinds

Of course not every case of a problem in the spine is so dramatic. Very often the owners of dogs, cats or horses tell us that their pet "somehow moves strangely" or "doesn't want to move properly". The dog doesn't want to lie down and even sitting down is painful. The cat no longer jumps onto the sofa or the horse is less smooth when riding. Also livestock and here, in particular, bulls often have back problems which are very frustrating as they

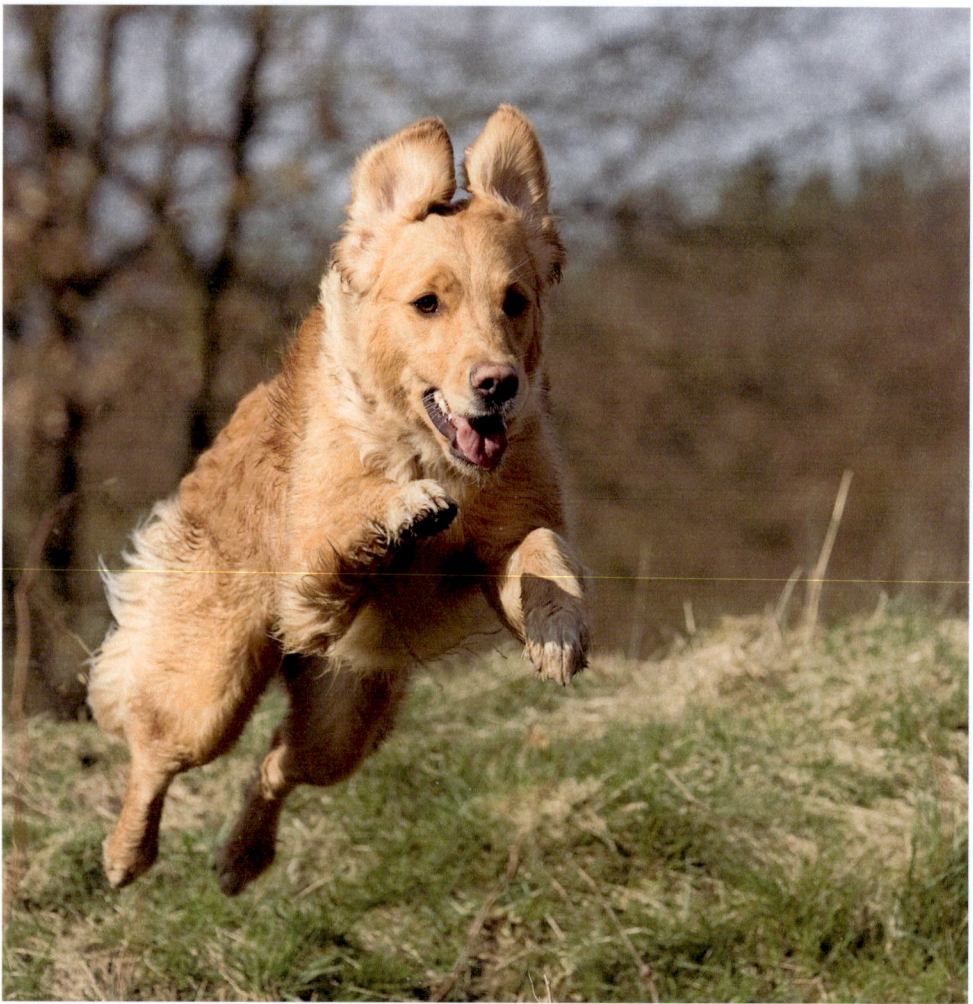

He is full of beans after his therapy.

reduce the stud service business and hence cause a great financial loss to the owner. In many cases the problems are not so acute and the owner has already seen other therapists or has tried to restore their pet's health with various compounds or with rest.

At the end of the day, most back problems result from blocks in the nerves' energy flow which needs to be restored. These blocks result in varying degrees of pain which then leads to a change in the patient's posture and hence often also to repositioning of the discs that can sometimes be made visible on an X-ray. Furthermore resulting problems can later also be found in gonarthrosis, hip arthrosis or diseases of the shoulder or the elbow joint. Many back problems in the area of the upper cervical spine originated in an unfavourable position of the foetus in the womb. Many back problems in equestrian sports, however, result from massive problems in the temporomandibular joint.

Fortunately most back problems can be treated quickly and with lasting effect with bioresonance. Programs for unblocking the vertebra as well as anti-inflammatory programs help us just as much as those for activating the lymph and toxin elimination which then have a positive influence on eliminating inflammatory substances. It is amazingly simple and quick to counteract the disease with the relevant frequencies and to restore working cell regulation and hence the energy flow of the neural pathways.

In isolated cases the general frequency programs might only bring about an improvement but not definite final healing. In these cases the organism is often severely infected with bacteria, viruses or fungi. In particular all back problems require special attention to be paid to infection of the organism with herpes viruses, Borrelia viruses, E. coli, Clostridials, Candida (neurotoxic) as well as Toxoplasma. Here, too bioresonance and its ability to transfer the relevant inverted oscillation[7] for the specific problem is a quick and effective way to heal those cases that are often considered irreparable in conventional medicine.

i. Autoimmune diseases

In the course of the last few years the so-called autoimmune diseases have also been on the rise in vet practices. The body does not develop antibodies against pollen, viruses, bacteria or parasites but against its own tissue. Scientists assume that an exogenous substance has a similar structure to a body's own tissue so that the antibodies produced not only fight the

---

[7] inverted oscillation: a mirror-imaged frequency pattern rotated 180°

responsible substance but also the body tissue. In human medicine diseases like Crohn's disease, a certain form of thyroiditis, lupus erythematosus as well as rheumatoid diseases are considered autoimmune diseases. Even multiple sclerosis is connected to an autoimmune reaction.

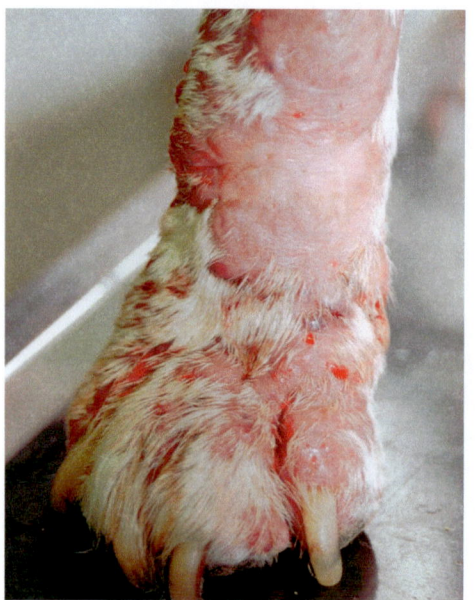

This bull terrier came with the conventional diagnosis of an autoimmune disease caused by massive bacterial infection.

In veterinary medicine we mainly see pemphigus and lupus in our dogs. In addition we must also check each hypothyroidism, in particular, with regard to the existence of antibodies to the thyroid tissue. Should those antibodies substantiate, they will destroy the thyroid tissue and will finally also lead to a hypo function of the thyroid. All these autoimmune diseases are mainly seen in predisposed breeds and genetic misinformation is held responsible for the emergence of these complexes.

Bioresonance will help to reveal manifold infections with viruses, fungi and bacteria and contamination with heavy metals that have accumulated over the course of the years and which the owner might not have noticed at the early stage. But now, when the first signs of these auto aggressive diseases appear, it is the last straw that breaks the camel's back and clinical symptoms, here mostly skin alterations, become visible. The aim of bioresonance therapy now is to eliminate all substances that pollute the organism and hence restore the healthy oscillation pattern of the body. However, in many cases, the problems caused by the number of stresses are so great that bioresonance leads to a significant improvement but cannot always achieve complete healing. The stresses can no longer be tested as pathological oscillation patterns. The disease persists, although in a diminished form.

Diagnosis with the Bicom optima

The bioresonance method offers the following solution with the Bicom optima: with

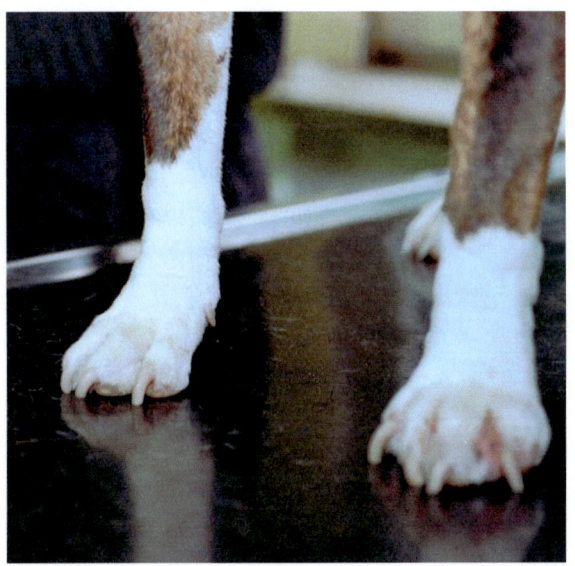

The same dog as in the previous picture - after three treatments with Bicom optima.

the help of a frequency pass we are able to energetically test the suitable frequency. In doing so, we are no longer testing programs but we are looking for individual oscillation patterns that resonate with the body and hence contain the missing key for healing. An experienced therapist will not give up until they find the patterns that caused the disease initially to appear not to be fully curable. Of course there are individual cases of animals that cannot be fully healed but we always have to be aware that bioresonance depends upon an organism that is able to respond. We can only heal by modulating a pathological oscillation pattern while there is reactive tissue.

j. Diseases of the oral cavity - diseases of the gums and teeth

Cats, especially, very often manifest a very painful disease of the mouth cavity, namely gingivitis stomatitis. The whole oral cavity of the cat exhibits severe inflammation in the area of the gums, which continues into the whole jaw angle and the oropharynx, partly with bloody open wounds. The clinical symptoms of this brutal disease are a refusal to eat, obvious symptoms of pain, increased dribbling and extremely bad breath. In addition we often find a further complex of symptoms in these cats, FORL – feline odontoclastic resorptive lesion. Many people equate FORL with cervical caries because all of a sudden the pulp in the area of the cervix of the teeth is exposed. However this is wrong as, in contrast to cervical caries in human beings, the pulp does not open from the mouth cavity but from the root – the tooth starts to dissolve from the root towards the top of the tooth.

While various studies have linked the development of FORL with abnormal information in the calcium / phosphorus metabolism and hence with an abnormal reaction of the osteoclasts, faucitis, as gingivitis stomatitis is also called due to its main location in the jaw angle, is obviously caused by various viral infections. In isolated cases they may even be found in biopsies of the mucous membranes.

Energetically speaking the gums belong to the stomach meridian, which is also affected in almost 90% of all cases of this disease. Bioresonance will help us to find out whether the problem is feeding the cat with kibble, which must be considered rather warm food in terms of energy, or whether the stomach meridian is affected by stress. However we must not neglect infection with fungi, namely Candida.

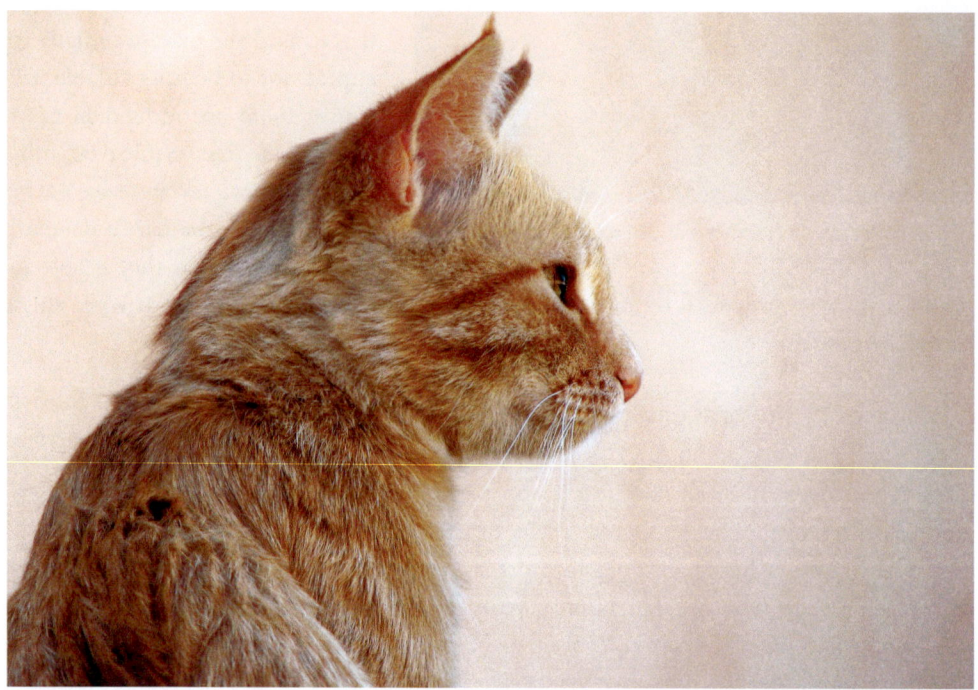

Therapeutic approach with Bicom optima

In most cases it is possible to stop the severe inflammation and bring about an alleviation of the cat's suffering by stabilizing the stomach meridian and eliminating the stresses found. However, as we are considering an autoimmune component in extreme cases, I have positive experience in my own practice of autohaemotherapy along with the general

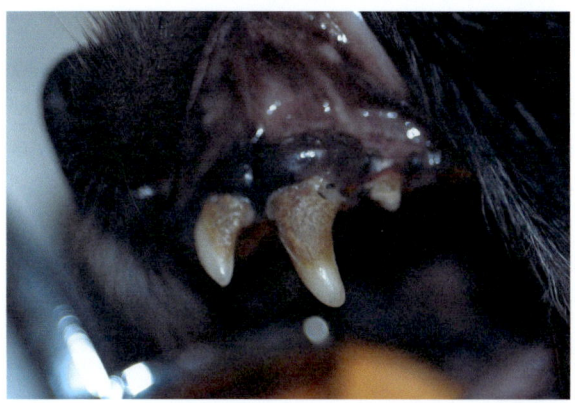

Excessive tartar indicates a disturbed energetic situation to the holistic therapist.

programs for activating the lymph system, toxin elimination and, of course, elimination of stresses.

The Bicom optima offers a predefined program so that we can do without the complex preparation of the blood that is necessary in conventional medicine. The pathological oscillation pattern is contained in each drop of blood. If you put a drop of blood into the input bowl, the bioresonance device is able to modulate a therapeutically effective oscillation pattern. In the majority of cases I have been able to achieve a significant reduction in the inflammation solely with bioresonance and only in few individual cases did we fail to produce a complete cure. But here again we must point out that a complete recovery requires reactive tissue.

Obstacles on the way to recovery – blocks

The energetic basic program of the Bicom optima alone and activation of the deficient eliminating organs will not always bring complete success, especially with chronic diseases. Although a significant improvement can be seen in these cases as well, we do not achieve final recovery. The solution in these persistent cases is to search for the so-called therapy blocks.

Mainly blocks caused by scars, energetic interference fields in teeth, geopathic stress, blocks of the lingual bone and the jaw joint as well as blocks of the sympathetic chain in the neck are considered as main therapy blocks.

Significance of scars

Speaking of scars, it is those that have occurred due to slow-healing wounds that are of great importance. For instance I can recall a horse that suffered from chronic bronchitis that did not fully heal until I dealt with an abnormal scar on the inside of the front leg in the area of the pisiform bone. Those therapists with experience in acupuncture will know that the lung meridian is located in this area and, upon testing with bioresonance and the 5 element test kit, this meridian proved to be in disorder – even without any knowledge of acupuncture.

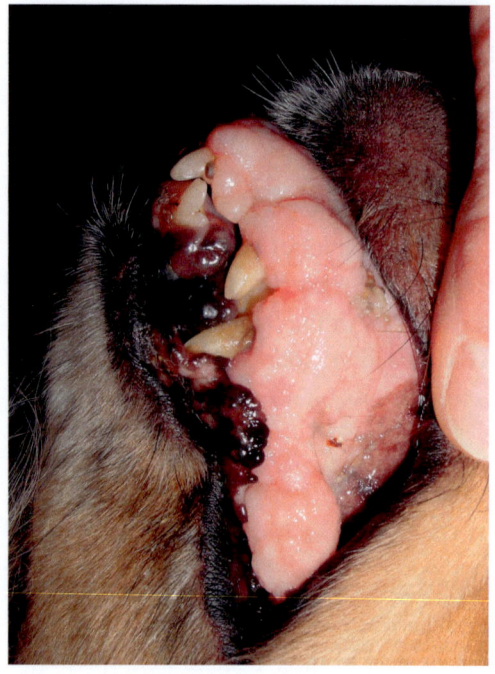

One of the reasons for such massive tumours in many cases are tooth interference fields that block healing and must be treated with bioresonance.

In energetic examination we are in the fortunate position that we don't have to rely on information given by owners with regard to existing scars, but we can test with pre-stored programs in the device whether a scar interference field exists. In many cases therapy with these programs will basically be sufficient to cancel the interfering effect. Only in very persistent cases in which the scar interference field appears time and time again when retesting, will we have to search the body for the exact location. This search will then be performed with the abovementioned magnetic depth probe, which is connected to the tensor and which helps us to locate the interference field.

If the organism does not resonate with the area examined with the depth probe, an interference field is located at that spot. Furthermore we can also examine individual teeth or the jaw joint, the sympathetic chain in the neck and the lingual bone with the help of a finger-shaped gold-plated electrode (gold finger) connected to the tensor. These areas can cause massive energetic interference fields, both in their own area and also in the organism as a whole, so that they may also cause pathological symptoms far away from the areas under examination.

For instance you may test the area of the root of the canines, which very often react in dogs with diseases of the hip joint. In all those interference fields we may find a hint either via pre-stored programs in the Bicom optima or via the relevant test technique with the 5-element test kit. Only if there are hints to existing interference fields, do we have to further clarify the exact location of this interference field in order to achieve complete success with the local bioresonance treatment of the problem area in cases where the therapy is delayed.

Radiation stress

My experience with geopathic and radiation stress, however, is slightly different. This comprises not only radiation stress caused by electronic smog, radioactivity and radio waves but of course also problems in the sense of watercourses running near where animals sleep or WLAN devices that we can hardly do without today, as well as TV sets that keep running in stand-by-mode and hence create electronic smog. Of course we are able to repair this interference in the body, but it can't be denied that if the source still exists, it will certainly cause new problems.

For instance I remember a horse in Spain with extreme skin alterations in the area of the croup and the legs. Testing revealed that the therapy block was electronic smog. Therapy then led to a marked improvement after three sessions at weekly intervals. Unfortunately the following re-testing still showed electronic smog. Only repeated therapy of the block and relocation of the horse into a different stable without any high-voltage lines crossing the building finally led to success.

Heavy metal

Another important issue when treating animals is checking possible contamination with heavy metal. Of course we will hardly find amalgam fillings in animals, but energetic mercury contamination is not uncommon. Possible causes for this may, on the one hand, be contamination of the feedstuff but also environmental pollution of the soil. Our chronic allergy patients, in particular, often display mercury contamination but chronic lameness in horses is also often associated with mercury contamination.

However I also recall a Frisian horse that had been suffering from an exudative suppurative inflammation of the hoof bulb, also called malanders, for 18 months. He had been treated with conventional medicine without success and the test revealed contamination with tin. After this was eliminated, the horse was free of symptoms and still is today – one year later – despite very damp conditions in the stable. The whys and wherefores of such heavy metal contamination cannot in most cases be reliably reproduced; for instance we cannot exclude the suspicion that contamination might have already occurred with a previous owner of the horse.

In my opinion these examples make very clear that initial success followed by a step backwards must not be equated to or associated with a failure of bioresonance. Every method is as good as its user and, in persistent cases like this, the therapist must be willing to record the "crime scene" of the patient like a detective and to reassess their approach and their therapy time and time again until they have finally found and treated the block.

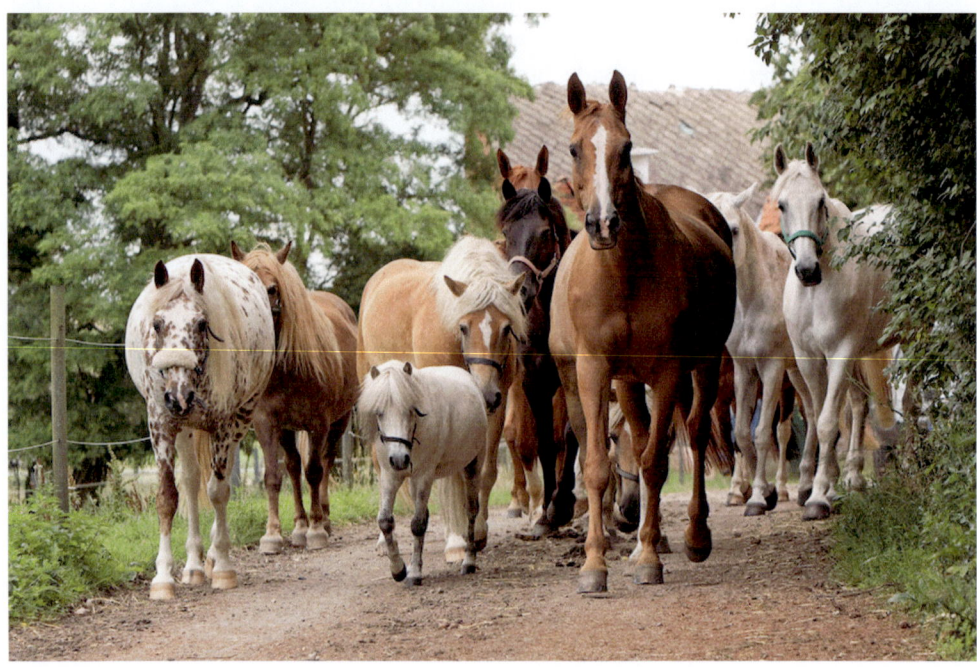

A healthy and relaxed herd of horses.

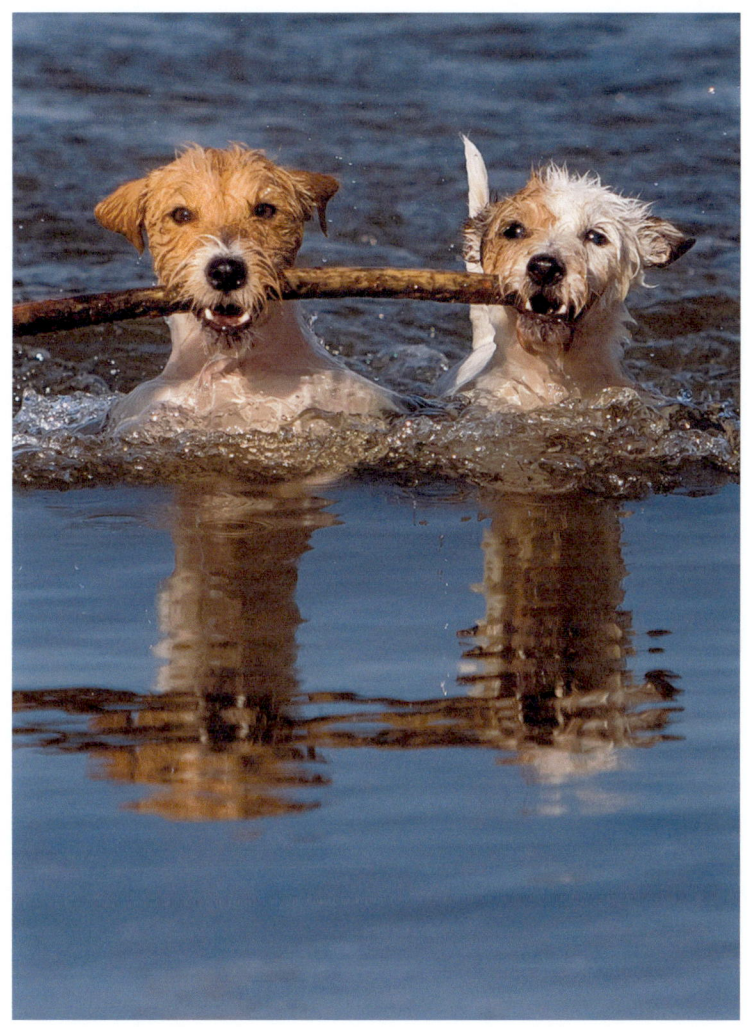

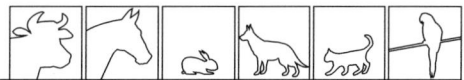

Additional possibilities with bioresonance

Based on the previous chapter about therapy blocks, it would be remiss not to tell you about further possibilities in bioresonance.

Nosodes in veterinary medicine and homeopathic potentiation with the Bicom optima

Colleagues experienced in natural medicine know about the effectiveness of nosodes with certain diseases. What are nosodes? They are germs that have been potentiated and that are used to encourage the body to regulate itself against these pathogens. "Let like cure like" was one of the principles of Samuel Hahnemann, the founder of homeopathy. Hahnemann also used potentiated substances to cause the organism to self-regulate and to heal his patients. While in the previous chapter we utilised the oscillation in the body and its modulation, we can equally well use the oscillation pattern of the secretion from a fistula, for instance, to directly apply it for therapy. To do so the potentiating program of the Bicom optima applies a nosode-like frequency pattern of the secretion, enabling the body to react specifically to the triggering noxa and hence to fight the disease.

Talking about oscillation patterns and secretions, we must also understand that everything on planet earth consists of a material part on the one hand and an energetic part on the other hand, both of which are characterized by a frequency or oscillation pattern. As the bioresonance method enables us to test these oscillation patterns directly on the patient, we are also able to test exactly how these substances should be applied. It is only logical that the particular requirements of each and every substance can be tested and applied for each patient.

A patient who resonates with the oscillation of an allopathic compound wants to be treated with the specific oscillation tested. Bioresonance even makes it very easy to test in advance whether or not a medicine will lead to the desired success in this particular patient.

In the case of mastitis we may, for instance, test which medicine will produce a cure. We might, of course, also treat such a disease with bioresonance to avoid any "down times" for the cow due to unusable milk. And, of course, the cow will show its gratitude with a significantly improved state of health. Foodstuff testing must be seen in the same context – pet owners' questions regarding the best possible food for their friends are no longer a problem for vets working with bioresonance. Those of you who start trying this procedure with bioresonance in your own practice will be surprised by the results.

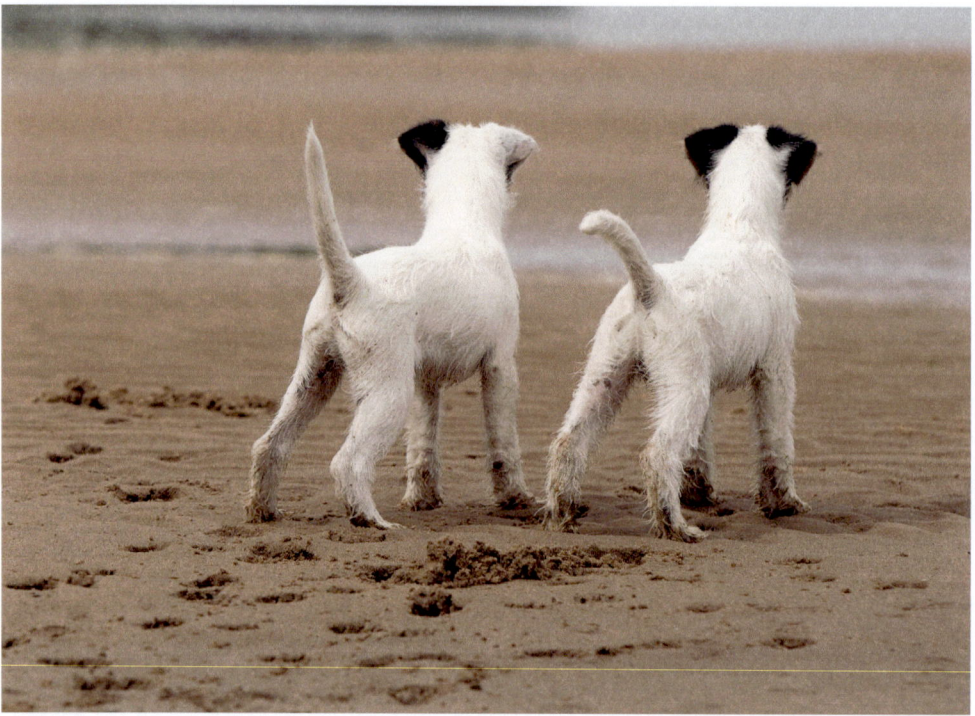

Two healthy young dogs - looking ahead into a bright future.

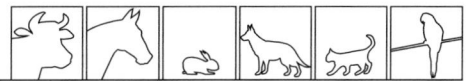

The evidence behind Bicom bioresonance

When bioresonance therapy was still in its infancy and, right from the outset, was achieving considerable success in healing and improving the quality of life of suffering patients, the critics excelled themselves with polemic reactions. They could not grasp that bodily functions can be activated by electromagnetic therapy. It was something which just did not seem to fit into their view of the world at all.

The effectiveness studies which were put forward were immediately pulled to pieces without any reasoned argument. Case studies were argued away with the famous placebo effect and significant scientific studies connected with bioresonance were simply ignored.

The following is a concise summary of the most important studies and reports.

Pre-clinical studies

Preclinical studies alone show that Bicom bioresonance therapy cannot possibly be based on a placebo effect. They also support the results of non-placebo-controlled cohort studies which are described later.

An initial study was conducted to determine whether the Bicom device could actually have an effect on biological systems. Tests on 50,000 blood samples and with several hundred settings proved, beyond any doubt, that the Bicom device affects biological systems in a manner which can be measured objectively. The phagocytosis activity of donor blood was significantly improved at certain settings.[8]

In another study Drosophila larvae were exposed to heat shock. The aim was to test whether the vitality of the Drosophila larvae damaged in this way could be restored using bioresonance. The results of this study show that the immune system of the Drosophila larvae could be improved and restored by transferring weak endogenous electromagnetic frequencies with the Bicom device, seen for example in the increase in survival times without food and normalisation of mobility.

---

8 O. Osadscha et al. at the R.E. Kavetzky Institute for Experimental Pathology, Oncology and Radiology of the State Academy of Sciences of the Ukraine, Kiev.

Another preclinical study dealt with the influence of Bicom bioresonance therapy on the structural dynamics of the serum albumin of patients with breast cancer. It was possible to demonstrate in an in vitro experiment that biological information in the HSA of healthy subjects could be transferred with the device to the HSA of cancer patients. Moreover, the self-regulatory processes of the immune system were restored and stable conformational change was achieved.[9]

An interesting study involved transferring information from acetic acid to mineral salt solutions with Bicom. The pH of the mineral salt solution dropped significantly as a result of this information transfer. Kirlian photography revealed marked differences in corona formation between informed and not informed samples and clear differences could also be observed in the development of structure in crystal formation.[10]

The last study to be mentioned in this series concerns transferring a toxic concentrated thyroxin solution to aquarium water with the bioresonance device. "This study demonstrated, through two double blind trails conducted independently of one another in Austria and Italy, that bioinformation can be scanned and transferred by the Bicom device. By transferring information from a concentrated toxic solution of the hormone thyroxin into aquarium water, the metamorphosis of tadpoles was slowed down markedly in numerous parallel experiments."[11]

Studies on treating allergy

The numerous studies on treating allergies and associated disease patterns provide conclusive proof of the effectiveness of Bicom bioresonance therapy. Admittedly they were conducted solely in human medicine but they are also applicable to animals. Since man is a mammal, as are most of our pets, use, response and results can certainly be transferred to animals.

---

[9] 4. O.V. Zhalko-Titarenko et. al.: Der Einfluss der Bicom Resonanz-Therapie auf die strukturelle Dynamik des Serum-Albumins von Patientinnen mit Brustkrebs; Wissenschaftliche Studien [The influence of Bicom resonance therapy on the structural dynamics of the serum albumin of patients with breast cancer; scientific studies], page 24-37, Institut für Regulative Medizin, Gräfelfing, 1999.

[10] N. Rojko Vuga, Prof. A. Jeglic's research group: Untersuchung der Transduktion von Essigsäure-Information [Studies on the transduction of acetic acid information], Erfahrungsheilkunde no. 7/98

[11] P. C. Endler et al.: Übertragung von Molekül-Information mittel Bioresonanz-Gerät (BICOM) im Amphibien versuch [Transfer of molecular information using the bioresonance device (BICOM) in experiments on amphibians], Erfahrungsheilkunde no. 3/95

The first of these studies was carried out by P. Schumacher as a retrospective effectiveness study and published under the title "Biophysikalische Therapie der Allergien [Treating allergies biophysically]."[12] It included all the children treated for allergy within a 6-month period, regardless of age, sex, severity of the condition and diagnosis. There were 164 patients in total, some with multiple problems, resulting in 204 cases. Effectiveness was verified 5 months later by questionnaire. Of the 204 cases within the same period, 83 % were symptom-free and 11 % improved. 4.5 % reported no change and 1.5 % could not be assessed.

In another study by Dr Schumacher, also conducted within a 6-month period, the results of treating 115 subjects allergic to pollen were evaluated. Some patients were affected by several different types of pollen, resulting in 145 cases in total. Allergy to meadow grasses was detected in approx. 80% of patients. The remainder were spread between alder, willow, rye and birch. The treatment period ran from November 1990 to April 1991 and the results were verified by questionnaire in October 1991. 43.4 % were symptom-free, 15.9 % had improved significantly, 34.5 % showed a noticeable change and 6.2 % reported no change.[13]

Another allergy study with 232 cases, exclusively involving adults where responsiveness is often more difficult than in children, was conducted by Dr J. Hennecke. Of these 232 cases, 50.4 % were symptom-free, 34.1 % were improved and 15.5% reported no change.[14]

It is worth mentioning that the syndromes in the allergic disorders group react differently, as can be seen from the following table.

Allergic disorders	Patients	Symptom-free	Improved	No change
Skin diseases	68	39 = 58.0 %	21 = 30.0 %	8 = 12.0 %
Pruritis	20	7 = 35.0 %	10 = 50.0 %	3 = 16.0 %
Conjunctivitis	16	10 = 62.5 %	5 = 31.0 %	1 = 6.5 %
Intestinal disease	13	10 = 77.0 %	1 = 7.5 %	2 = 15.5 %

---

[12] Sonntag Verlag, Stuttgart, 1998, page 125-132.

[13] loc. cit., page 149-152.

[14] J. Hennecke: Zwei Jahre Erfahrung mit der meridianbezogenen Allergie-Therapie – Auswertung einer statistischen Studie [Two years' experience of meridian-based allergy therapy – evaluation of a statistical study] Ärztezeitschrift f. Naturhvf., 35 (6) 427-432, 94.

Allergic disorders	Patients	Symptom-free	Improved	No change
Respiratory tract diseases	46	19 = 41.5 %	21 = 45.5 %	6 = 13.0 %
Pollen allergy	69	32 = 47.0 %	21 = 31.0 %	16 = 23.0 %
Total	232	117 = 50.4 %	79 = 34.1 %	36 = 15.5 %

A number of Chinese doctors have carried out studies in various state hospitals with impressive results. Some of these are presented here in table form for convenience. They are an impressive endorsement of the abovementioned studies.

Author	Publication	Results
Yuan Ze, Huang Jiali, Wang Haiyan, Yu Chunyan – The Clinical Results of Bicom 2000; single group cohort study, N = 154	Report: Paediatric Department of Xi'an Central Hospital, postcode 710003	77.8 % recovery 11.1 % definite recovery 7.8 % effect 3.3 % no effect
Yuan Ze, M. D. and Wang Haiyan: Clinical results with the Bicom 2000 bioresonance device; Xi'an City Central Hospital, China; cohort study with follow-up N = 1639	Lecture: 45th International Congress for Bicom users, 29.4. to 1.5.2005, Fulda;	82.6 % recovery 8.8 % obviously effective 5.8 % effective 2.8 % ineffective
Du Xia, Liu Yuanxia and Yang Jinzhi: Clinical observation of 79 cases of allergic skin disease using the bioresonance device; single group cohort study N = 79	Certified translation: Chinese Journal of Practical Medicine, volume 4, no. 3, March 03	74.7 % recovery 15.2 % visible effect 7.6 % effective 2.5 % ineffective

Author	Publication	Results
Feng Yizhen, Chen Huanzhi, Li Ruifeng, Liu liping: Clinical observation of the healing effect of the bioresonance device in 150 cases of allergy in children	Certified translation: Chinese Journal of Current Paediatrics CJCP, June 2005, volume 7, no. 3	60.7 % recovery 34.0 % effective 5.3 % in effective
Song Ke-min, Yang Rong-ya, AO Jun-hong, Zhang Jie: The clinical study of Bicom allergy therapy	Journal of Clinical Dermatology, vol. 32, number 10, 2003;	46.7 % successful treatment (symptom-free) 23.3 % improvement 15.0 % reaction 15.0 % no reaction
Huan Shuiming, Sun Zhang-ping, Fang Yucai: Clinical observation of the treatment of allergic rhinoconjunctivitis and bronchial asthma in children with the bioresonance therapy device (Bicom) randomised controlled prosp. parallel group study N = 172	Zhe Jiang Medicine, Zhe Jiang Medical Journal, edition B, 2005, volume 27, Medical Association	**BICOM group:** 46.0 % marked effect 39.7 % effective 14.3 % in effective **following unsuccessful treatment with with medication** with Bicom 35.2 % marked effect 44.4 % effective 20.4 % ineffective **treatment solely with medication:** 32.7 % marked effect 36.4 % effective 30.9 % ineffective
Xu Minhong et al. Clinical observation of the treatment of chronic nettle rash with the bioresonance therapy device single group cohort study N = 56	Certified translation: Core Chinese Scientific Journal, Journal of Dermatology and Venereology, vol. 21, no. 7, July 2005	35.8 % recovery 25.0 % visibly effective 12.5 % effective 26.7 % in effective

Author	Publication	Results
Zhan Xinlian, Wang Wenjie, Liu Qiang: Clinical observation of 54 cases of nettle rash with the Bicom bioresonance device, single group cohort study N = 54	Certified translation: Core Scientific and Technical Journal of China	40.7 % recovery 25.9 % definite improvement 18.5 % effect 14.8 % no effect

I will end this section on allergy with one particularly impressive study. It was also conducted in China by Wang Jun and Lu Shu Jin and presented in 2006 at a congress in Fulda: "Klinische Studie der Therapie von allergischem Asthma und allergischer Rhinitis [Clinical study of treatment of allergic asthma and allergic rhinitis]." It was verified 6 months later. The results are also presented in table form for the sake of clarity.[15]

Allergic disorder	cases treated	no effect	effective	visible effect	recovery	recovery	recovery + visible effect
						in %	
Asthma	786	13	69	45	659	83.8	89.6
Rhinitis	593	16	19	52	506	85.3	95.1
Urticaria	387	18	37	46	286	73.9	85.8
Eczema, child	122	3	2	5	112	91.8	95.9
Eczema, adult	102	6	39	15	42	41.2	55.9
Neurodermatitis	86	10	17	12	47	54.7	68.7
Purpura	63	3	6	14	40	63.5	85.7
Conjunctivits	32	1	2	3	26	81.3	90.6
Solar dermatitis	12	1	2	1	8	66.7	90.6
Porokeratosis	3	1	1	0	1	33.3	75.0

---

[15] Congress proceedings RTI 30 of the International Medical Research Group on Bicom Bioresonance Therapy, 2006,

Allergic disorder	cases trea-ted	no effect	effective	visible effect	recovery	recovery	recovery + visible effect
						in %	
Total	2186	72	194	193	1727	-.-	-.-
		3 %	9 %	9 %	79 %	79 %	87.8 %

Studies of other indications

Studies dealing with other indications prove furthermore that the use of Bicom bioresonance is not limited to treating allergies. It would not be appropriate to describe Bicom therapy as a universal panacea yet experience shows that Bicom bioresonance therapy can be used with all indications, either on its own or as a preparatory, supporting or concluding treatment.

In 2006 a scientific survey involving a total of 541 case studies was carried out in 31 practices as a retrolective longitudinal cohort study. Analysis revealed that 43% of the indications surveyed had recovered, 48% had improved and 9% of cases treated showed no change.[16]

This gives rise to the following table when split according to syndromes.

Summarised outcome				All results as %
	Recovered	Improved	No change	Deteriorated
Acute + chronic infection	60	37	3	0
Respiratory tract diseases	42	50	8	0
Cardiovascular disorders	13	61	26	0
Auto-immune diseases	15	66	19	0
Tumours	35	48	13	4
Gastroenterological disorders	54	42	4	0

[16] Congress proceedings RTI 30 of the International Medical Research Group on Bicom Bioresonance Therapy, 2006, 46th International Congress.

	Recovered	Improved	No change	Deteriorated
Damage to the liver parenchyma	36	65	0	0
Degenerative disorders of the skeletal and locomotor system	33	57	10	0
Endocrinological disorders	38	54	8	0
Injuries and their consequences	69	23	8	0
Non-specific pain therapy	43	47	10	0
Menstrual problems	59	41	0	0
Dental problems	55	45	0	0

Outcome of all study indications	Recovered	Improved	No change	Deteriorated
Number of cases 541 =100 %	235	262	43	1
as %	43.4	48.4	8.0	0.2

Dr Machowinski, together with the University of Heidelberg, conducted a prospective randomised study to examine the success of treatment of hepatic dysfunction with patients' own electromagnetic fields (Bicom). 28 patients with slight chronic liver cell damage were treated.

After 12 weeks, analysis showed that GOT, GPT and gamma GT levels in the Bicom group were much improved compared with those of the comparison group. The levels in the comparison group showed no change.[17]

As part of their thesis B. J. Papez and Joze Barovic conducted a study to examine the effect of Bicom resonance therapy on excessive strain in top athletes.

Two groups each consisting of 12 top athletes with excessive strain syndrome were treated with conventional medicine and with Bicom. In summary, therapy time was shorter in

---

[17] Paper at the Congress in Fulda on 16 April 1996; Scientific Studies, Institut für Regulative Medizin, 1999, page 77-92

the Bicom group, fewer treatments were needed and there were no side effects.[18]

Dr Huff's naturopathic practice conducted a retrolective effectiveness study of mycosis therapy by means of the Bicom device. 439 patients with Candida were treated over a 3-year period. 93% were treated successfully. Only in 7% did a relapse occur.

Scientific studies

Finally to conclude this review, I will now take a look at basic research into bioresonance. Numerous scientific studies provide evidence that organisms, organ function, cell function and cell communication are all regulated by electromagnetic frequency patterns and that these can be used for therapeutic purposes.

The Americans H. S. Burr and F. S. C. Northrop drew attention to this phenomenon back in 1935. In the abstract to their work "The electro-dynamic theory of life" they write: "There are several factors which suggest that living things must be viewed from the electro-dynamic point of view... "Potential gradients and polar differences exist in living systems. If this is the case, then electro-dynamic fields are also present." ..."The pattern or organisation of every biological system is established by complex electromagnetic fields." "As well as establishing this, it must maintain behaviour patterns amidst physical and chemical fluctuation. As a result it has to regulate and control living things. It must be the mechanism, whose action represents completeness, organisation and continuity."[19]

Leon Glas of the Dept. of Physiology, Centre of Nonlinear Dynamics in Physiology and Medicine, McGill University of Montreal, Canada observes in a study that all biological oscillation phenomena are essentially attributable to nonlinear systems of coupled oscillators. This in turn means that the generally accepted and thoroughly researched laws of physics relating to nonlinear systems are valid. It follows directly from these laws that these systems can only be influenced to a meaningful degree by means of ultraweak signals. For only ultraweak signals, if introduced into the system at the right time, are capable of significantly altering these kinds of oscillation systems. Disease frequently causes the transition from normal to pathological rhythms.[20] It is precisely these laws which lie behind bioresonance therapy.

---

[18] Report: Maribor Teaching Hospital, Slovenia, Clinical Rehabilitation Dept.; EHK 1999, 48 (7) 449-450.

[19] The University of Chicago Press. vol. 10. no. 3 (Sept. 1935, pp 322-333.

[20] Synchronisation and Rhythmic Processes in Physiology, NATURE: 410/8) 277-284, 2001

K. Torgele et al., Austrian Universities' Atomic Institute, Photobiophysics Research Group, Vienna, write in the summary to their work Elektromagnetische Bioinformation [Electromagnetic bioinformation]: "Electromagnetic bioinformation is considered to be the synthesis of two fundamental phenomena of life. On the one hand, electromagnetic interaction is dominant in living organisms. All physiological processes are based upon it. Perception of surroundings is also inconceivable without electromagnetic interaction." …"Organisms obviously also have the ability to emit characteristic light themselves and to process this light as bioinformation."[21]

Alessandro Sergi, School of Physics, University of KwaZulu-Natal, SA, observes in his article "Quantum Biology": "Some quantum effects in biology are reviewed and quantum mechanics is acknowledged as conceptually important to biology since without it most (if not all) of the biological structures and signalling processes would not even exist. Moreover, it is suggested that long-range quantum coherent dynamics, including electron polarisation, may be invoked to explain signal amplification processes in biological systems in general."[22]

Finally I should like to quote K.J. Pienta und D.S. Coffey.[23] They write in the abstract to their report "Informationsübertragung zellulärer Schwingungsinformation über ein Gewebs-Tensegrity-Matrix-System [Cellular harmonic information transfer through a tissue tensegrity-matrix system]":

"Cells and intracellular elements are capable of vibrating in a dynamic manner with complex harmonics, the frequency of which can now be measured and analysed in a quantitative manner by Fourier analysis. …The vibrational interactions occur through a tissue matrix system, consisting of the nuclear matrix, the cytoskeleton, and the extracellular matrix, that is poised to couple the biologic oscillations of the cell from the peripheral membrane to the DNA through a tensegrity-matrix structure. Tensegrity has been defined as a structural system composed of discontinuous compression elements connected by continuous tension cables. A tensegrity tissue matrix system allows for specific transfer of information through the cell by direct transmission of vibrational chemomechanical energy through harmonic wave motion."

---

[21] Elektromagnetische Bioinformation – eine Übersicht [Electromagnetic bioinformation – a survey]: Forschende Komplementärmedizin, volume 2, issue 3, June 1905.

[22] Published in: Atti della Academia Peloritana dei Pericolanti Vol. LXXXVII, C1C0901001, 2009.

[23] Department of Urology and Centre for Oncology of Johns Hopkins University, School of Medicine, Baltimore, Maryland 21205, USA, quoted

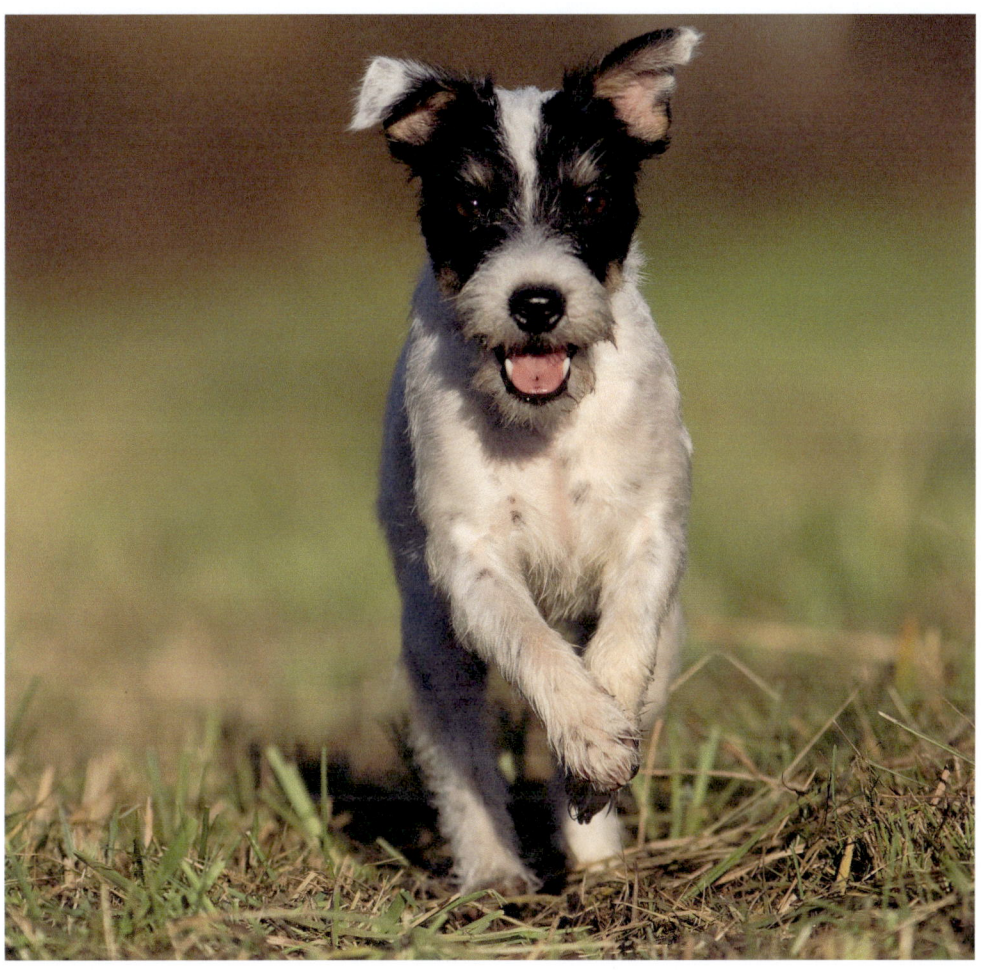